Chemistry of Essential Oils Made Even Simpler

By Michelle M. Truman, Ed.D.

Important Notice

This book is intended for informational purposes only. It is not provided in order to diagnose, prescribe, or treat any disease, illness, or injured condition of the body. The author, publisher, and printer accept no responsibility for such use. Anyone suffering from any disease, illness, or injury should consult with a physician or other appropriate licensed health care professional. In cases where inflammation may be present, exercise extreme caution in the application of essential oils on the skin.

Dedication

Dedicated to my dear husband, Brad Truman, who has been at my side for 27 years and has been with me through all of my educational pursuits and loves me in spite of my need to be a lifelong learner. Thank you for your love and support!

Acknowledgements

Many thanks to:

- Dr. David Stewart for helping me regain my spirituality and find the love (and understanding) of chemistry.

- Dr. Gary Young for the gift he has given us with these precious oils and the knowledge of how to use them.

- To Marnie Penkalski and Courtney Kaul for all their editing efforts. You ladies rock the grammar world!

- To Nancy Gouch and Carolyn Cooperman for their expertise in all things chemistry and oily. You two are such a pleasure to work with!

- To Penny Cosner for sharing her wonderful photos of the harvest!

- To my parents, Nial and Sally McClellan, for introducing me to these lovely companions...essential oils and for supporting me in all that I do.

- To my daughters, Aubrey and Tayler Truman, for putting up with their mom's education pursuits and loving me anyway. Xo
Thank you for taking many of the beautiful photos in this book!

♦Table of Contents

◆Why Do I Need to Know Chemistry?

Anyone can use essential oils, but if you can understand how they work in the body you can choose the oils that work the best for you, your family, and your friends.

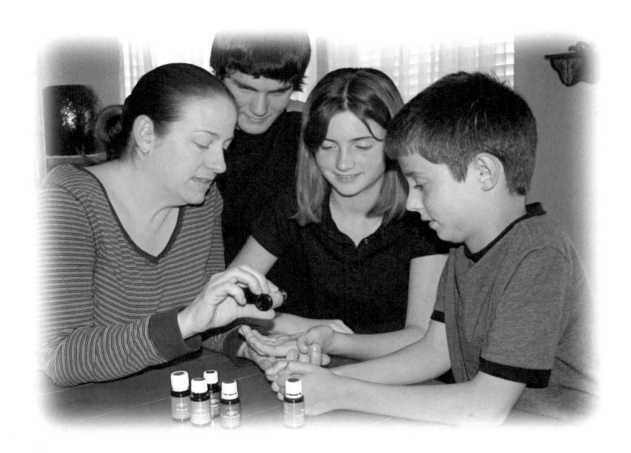

Another important thing to understand is that your belief in how the oils work has an effect on how well they perform. Adding science to faith is a benefit to you!

♦The Left and Right Brain Work Together

The left side of your brain is the reasoning and mathematical side while the right side of your brain is the intuitive or creative part. To fully understand what you will read in this book you need to use both your intuition and your reasoning sides together.

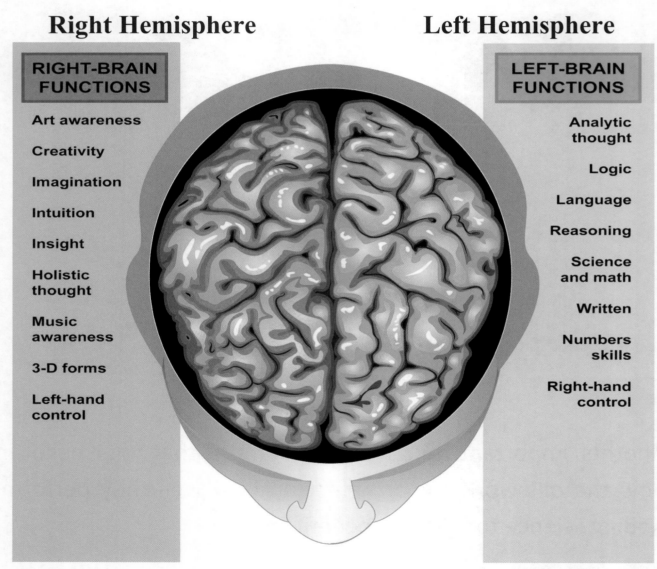

Right Hemisphere   **Left Hemisphere**

RIGHT-BRAIN FUNCTIONS	LEFT-BRAIN FUNCTIONS
Art awareness	Analytic thought
Creativity	Logic
Imagination	Language
Intuition	Reasoning
Insight	Science and math
Holistic thought	Written
Music awareness	Numbers skills
3-D forms	Right-hand control
Left-hand control	

"God is in the details." -Dr. David Stewart

♦Use Oils to Assist in Comprehension

Before you begin to read/study this book use the following oils to help give you courage, break mental blocks, and keep a clear head. These oils will help you understand the power and genius of the oils.

Oil	Reason	Place
Valor	For courage to learn chemistry	Wrists and breathe deeply
Cedarwood	To help remember what you learn	Right thumb and roof of mouth
Lemon	To increase alertness	Temples, forehead, and breathe deeply
Peppermint	To increase alertness	Neck, chest, and breathe deeply *(Don't get near your eyes!)*

◆Four Ways Essential Oils Get in the Body

One: Inhale

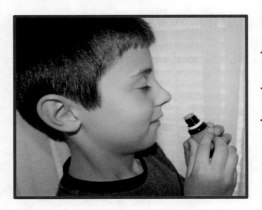

Breathe it through your nose to allow the tiny molecules of the oils to enter the blood stream through the lungs. They will proceed into the olfactory nerves in the middle of the brain. Inhale directly from the bottle, diffuse with a diffuser, or drop into your palm and breathe deeply.

Two: Skin

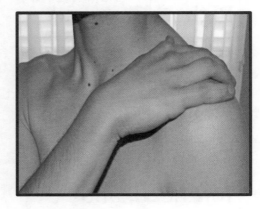

The skin is actually the largest organ in the body and is called the epidermis. The oil passes through the skin and goes directly into your cells to a place in the body where it is needed. You can drop the oil directly from the bottle onto the place you would like the oil to target or you can place a couple drops in your hand, rub your palms together, and massage onto a location.

NOTE: Oils can sometimes be irritating to the skin. If irritation does occur apply an organic vegetable oil to the skin (V6). Do NOT apply water as it will push the oil deeper into the skin.

Three: Swallowing

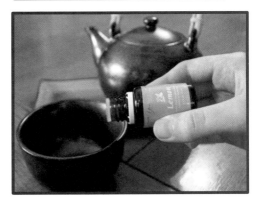

You can put essential oils into clear vegetable capsules and swallow, add to liquids and drink, drop directly on the tongue and swallow, or use for flavor when cooking meals.

Four: Body Orifices

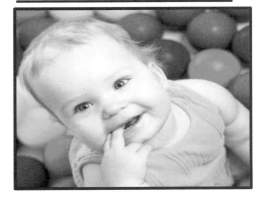

Rub the selected oil inside the mouth, under the tongue, or inside the cheeks without swallowing. Suppositories can be used and the oil can be directly absorbed by the lining of the rectum.

Every 'body' is different. What works for one person may not work for another. It is best to use the oils, get familiar with them, become friends with them. There are tools to assist us in the healing process.

- Essential Oils Desk Reference
  by Life Science Publishing

- Reference Guide for Essential Oils
  by Connie and Alan Higley

◆How are Essential Oils Used?

There are three perspectives: German, British, and French.

The **British** believe that all essential oils should be diluted in a fatty oil and that no more than 5% of the mixture should be essential oils. They usually use essential oils in massage therapy.

The British also believe that aromatherapy can be unsafe because most oils are not at a quality that is safe for undiluted applications.

The **Germans** believe in the aroma of the oils. This is where the term 'aromatherapy' originated.

Their perspective is that the molecules of the oils will be taken directly into the brain through the olfactory nerves which are connected to the middle of the brain.

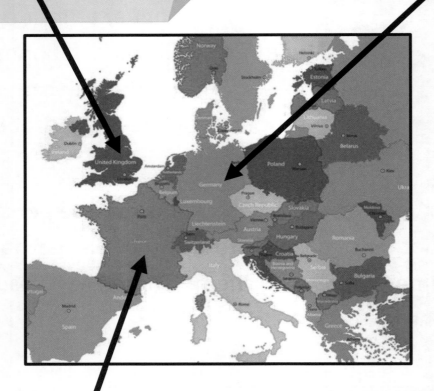

The **French** believe in all four methods of taking oil into the body: inhale, skin, swallow, and body orifices; therefore, they also know that oils need to be therapeutic grade.

They believe that the emphasis should be on the 'therapy', not just the 'aroma' as in the German perspective.

The **French** perspective is the perspective Gary Young of Young Living Essential Oils and other knowledgeable doctors in the field of aromatherapy say is the correct perspective from which to use the oils. They are safe if we use a "common sense" approach to their usage.

◗Essential Oils in the United States

In the United States there are <u>no</u> standards for therapeutic grade essential oils set by any government agency.

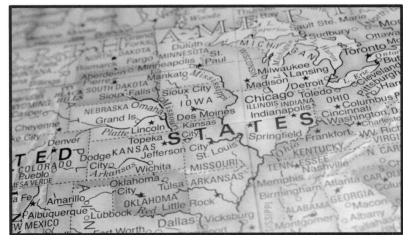

The French have an agency called AFNOR (*Association Francaise de Normalization*) that regulates the quality of French products and sets standards for oils.

The ISO (International Standardization Organization) in Geneva, Switzerland has adopted the ANFOR standards for oils as the international standard. However, these standards are just a set of minimums. It does not matter if the ingredients of the oil being tested are grown naturally or created in a lab by scientists. The oils are certified as long as they meet the minimum standard.

Young Living's standards are higher than AFNOR or ISO. They test every batch of oil to see if it meets Young Living's own standards and if it does not, it is discarded or returned to the supplier.

⬥Growing a Therapeutic Grade Essential Oil

First, start with a perfect seed that has been identified by experts as the correct species.

Second, plant the seed in clean soil without any chemicals. If you grow a plant in soils filled with chemicals, those chemicals will be transferred to the plant and finally into your body.

Third, harvest the plant at the peak of its oil producing cycle.

This is something **Young Living** does well on its own farms located in:

- *Mona, Utah, U.S.*
- *St. Maries, Idaho, U.S.*
- *Simiane-la-Rotonde, France*
- *Oman*
- *Guayaquil, Ecuador*

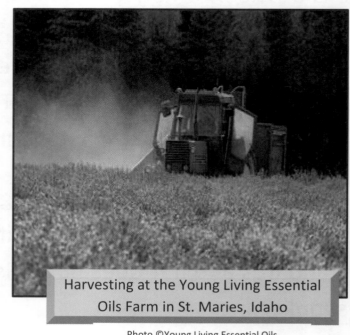

Harvesting at the Young Living Essential Oils Farm in St. Maries, Idaho

Photo ©Young Living Essential Oils

8

Fourth, distill the oil using low-temperatures and low-pressure steam distillation. This keeps all the healthy plant compounds in every batch of oil. This cannot be done quickly with high temperatures without killing the 'energy' of the oil.

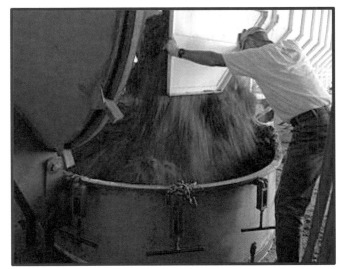

Distiller at Young Living Farms
Photo ©Young Living Essential Oils

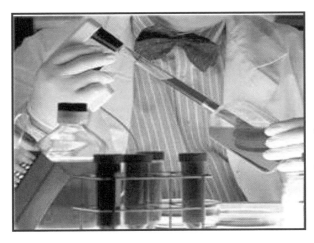

Fifth, the oil is placed into dark amber bottles to protect it from heat and light. Some of the oil is then sent to a lab. The lab tests the oil to make sure it meets and exceeds all requirements.

Sixth, the bottles are wrapped with labels that show exactly what is in the bottle including the genus and species. Not all companies do this.

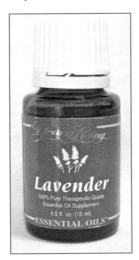

Details on what is in the bottle:

Genus: Lavandula
The genus is a major subdivision of a family or subfamily in the classification of organisms, usually consisting of more than one species.

Species: angustifolia
A subdivision of a genus or subgenus, the basic category of biological classification, made up of related individuals that resemble one another.

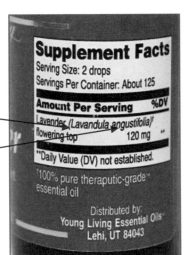

Supplement Facts
Serving Size: 2 drops
Servings Per Container: About 125

Amount Per Serving   %DV
Lavender (Lavandula angustifolia)
flowering top   120 mg   **

**Daily Value (DV) not established.

100% pure theraputic-grade™ essential oil

Distributed by:
Young Living Essential Oils™
Lehi, UT 84043

♦Are all Oils Created Equally?

There are three types of essential oils: fragrance, food, and therapeutic grade. 95% of all essential oils are made for the food and fragrance industries.

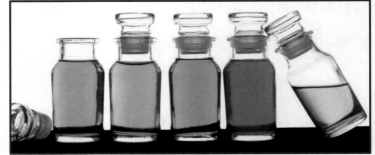

There are hundreds of ingredients that make-up a pure therapeutic grade essential oil, but not all oils are used for healing or therapeutic purposes.

Fragrance Grade	Food Grade	Therapeutic Grade
The fragrance industry is interested in *just* the ingredients that give things a nice smell. In a lab, they remove those ingredients and use them in their perfumes, make-up, lotions, etc.	The flavor industry is interested in *just* the ingredients that give things their flavor. In the lab, they take out the ingredients that taste like mint, cinnamon, wintergreen, and peppermint and use those small amounts to make mints, gum, mouthwash, etc.	There are hundreds of ingredients that make-up a natural essential oil. All the ingredients combined together in the essential oil are responsible for the healing that occurs when you use them. If an ingredient is missing the oil will not work because something important is gone.

♦Example of a Food Grade Oil

A food grade oil is added to spearmint gum to give it the spearmint flavor. It has been made in a lab so that every batch of spearmint gum tastes the same.

Gum is created with a base of plastics and rubber; then the manufacture adds in synthetic color and *flavor*. When they begin mixing, they add the synthetic sweeteners.

To watch this process go to youtube.com and search "How is chewing gum made".

Wrigley's Spearmint Gum Nutrition Information

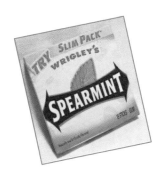

Nutrition Facts
Serving Size 1 stick (2.7g)
Calories 10

Amount/Serving	%DV*
Total Fat 0g	0%
Sodium 0mg	0%
Total Carbohydrate 2g	1%
Sugars 2g	
Protein 0g	

* Percent Daily Values (DV) are based on a 2,000 calorie diet.

INGREDIENTS: SUGAR, GUM BASE, DEXTROSE, CORN SYRUP; LESS THAN 2% OF: *NATURAL AND ARTIFICIAL FLAVORS*, GLYEROL, SOY LECITHIN, ASPARTAME, ACESULFAME K, COLORS (YELLOW 5 LAKE, BLUE 1 LAKE), BHT (TO MAINTAIN FRESHNESS). **PHENYLKETONURICS: CONTAINS PHENYLALANINE.**

(retrieved July 10, 2011 from http://www.wrigley.com/global/brands/spearmint.aspx#panel-3)

Synthetic spearmint created in a lab and used to flavor gum does not have any healing capabilities.

♦Synthetic vs. Therapeutic Essential Oils

To have a truly therapeutic grade oil we know it must start with the perfect seed, planted in clean soil, harvested at peak time, and distilled at a low-temperature and low-pressure, and all the inherent ingredients of the oil must be present.

What do we know about how synthetic oils are created?

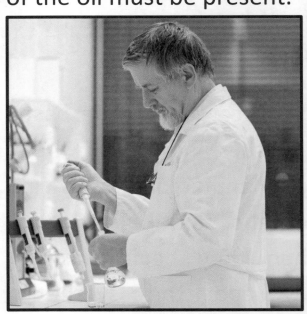

Scientists in labs have machines called '*gas chromatographs*' and use them to identify ingredients that make-up an essential oil. These are called 'formulas'. Scientists take the naturally occurring formula, change it, create it in a lab and make what they call a 'synthetic' version.

Dictionary.com states that synthetic means:
> "*pertaining to compounds formed through a chemical process by human agency, as opposed to those of natural origin.*"

Something we could call imitation!

♦Synthetics Do Not Heal

The process of taking something natural and recreating it in a lab would change the original way God created it. He created it to work perfectly in your body; the synthetic version does not do the same healing work in your body.

Something else to think about is that even though we live in a highly technological age, we do not yet have advanced enough technology to identify all the ingredients in essential oils. Scientists call these unknown ingredients *'constituents'* which means *'a part of something'*.

If we don't even know all the *'ingredients'* of the oils, but try to recreate them in a lab, it stands to reason that they would be missing essential parts of the nature made oil. Some of those parts may be just the ones that are needed for healing!

God Almighty first planted a garden. And indeed it is the purest of human pleasures.

-- Francis Bacon 1561-1626

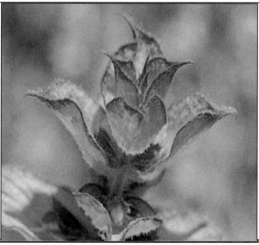

Clary sage (*Salvia sclarea*) in bloom at a Young Living's farm before being harvested for clary sage essential oil.

Photo ©Young Living Essential Oils

♦What Exactly is an Essential Oil?

Essential oils are the life blood of a plant; they circulate through tissues and pass through cell walls, carrying nutrition into the cells and carrying waste products out.

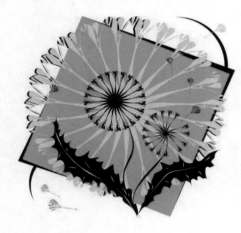

Have you ever broken a dandelion stem and felt the fluid drain on your fingers?

That is the fluid of the plant helping it to survive and live a healthy life.

The essential oils can be distilled out of many parts of a plant: *stems, branches, fruits, flowers, seeds, roots, bark, needles, and leaves.*

Scientists have identified hundreds of compounds found in essential oils. An example is Orange oil. It has hundreds of compounds including: alcohols, esters, aldehydes, ketones, carboxylic acids, and terpenes. However, there are compounds that have not been found yet so there could be many more!

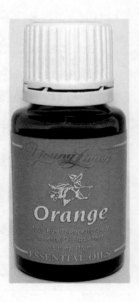

♦Essential Oils and Fatty Oils

Plants potentially produce two types of oils: fatty oil and essential oil.

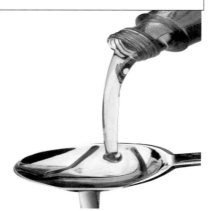

- Essential oils are found throughout the plant in the roots, stems, leaves, seeds, flowers, branches, etc.
- Fatty oils come from the seeds of plants. Fatty oils are called vegetable, base, or carrier oils.

Essential Oils	Fatty Oils
1. Distilled from plant parts	1. Processed from seeds
2. Not involved with seed *germination* and early growth	2. Necessary food for seeds to *germinate* and spout
3. Essential to the life processes of the plant	3. Not essential to the life processes of the plant
4. Tiny molecules	4. Large molecules
5. Molecules built from rings and short chains	5. Molecules built from long chains (larger molecular size)
6. Aromatic and volatile	6. Nonaromatic and nonvolatile
7. Circulate throughout the plants and in human bodies	7. Do not circulate in plants or in human bodies
8. Can pass through tissues, cell walls, and cell membranes	8. Do not pass through tissues, cell walls, or cell membranes
9. Not greasy to the touch	9. Greasy to the touch
10. Do not spoil or turn rancid	10. Can spoil and turn rancid
11. Antibacterial, antiviral, antifungal, antiphrastic, antiseptic	11. Not antibacterial, antiviral, antifungal, antiphrastic, antiseptic

(Table from <u>The Chemistry of Essential Oils Made Simple</u>, David Stewart, 2005, p. 55)

♦What is Homeostasis?

Homeostasis is defined by Webster's Online dictionary as: *"The processes whereby the internal environment of an organism tends to remain balanced and stable."* Dr. Stewart refers to this as *"a state of perfect wellness."* (p. 59)

When essential oils are applied to people, they do much or the same tasks as they do in plants. They circulate through the tissues and pass through the cell walls, carrying nutrition into the cells and removing waste products.

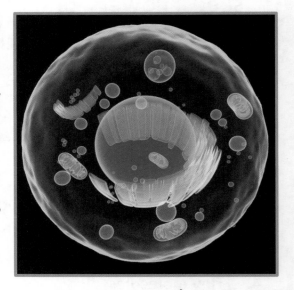

Essential oils work in our bodies to restore and maintain balance by cleansing the receptor sites of the cells of things that disrupt their proper function such as drugs (pharmaceutical, over the counter, and recreational), heavy metals, toxins, and petrochemicals.

This means that the daily usage of therapeutic grade essential oils has the potential to fight off dis-eases in bodies and help keep us well.

◆Essential Oils bring the body back into Balance or Homeostasis

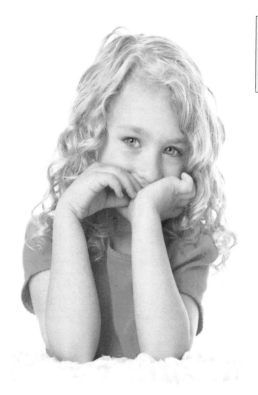

Think of **Goldilocks:** *Not too much... Not too little...It is just right!*

The oil of Myrtle can stimulate an increase or decrease in thyroid activity and bring the body back into balance. It is an adaptogen, meaning it is able to adapt to what the body needs to promote or restore normal function or homeostasis.

Therapeutic grade essential oils have intelligent discrimination to do what the body needs them to do.

On the other hand, drugs are created in a lab for one purpose, no matter what the body needs. They act as robots, preprogrammed to do what the drug makers tell them to do.

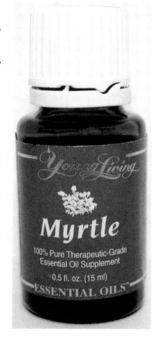

♦What is Chemistry?

Chemistry is the study of matter. Matter is anything that has mass and takes up space. Every human has mass and so our bodies are made up of matter.

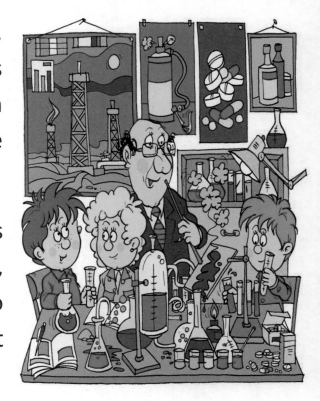

There are three types of particles that make-up matter: electrons, protons, and neutrons. They are so small that scientists have to look at them under powerful microscopes.

- Electrons = e- (have a negative charge)
- Protons = p+ (have a positive charge)
- Neutrons= n (are neutral so no charge)

If you mix electrons (e-), protons (p+), and neutrons (n) together you have an atom.

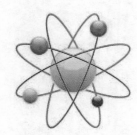

ChemCool.com defines an atom as:

"The smallest object that retains properties of an element, composed of electrons and a nucleus (containing protons and neutrons)."

♦Basic Chemistry

When electrons, protons, and neutrons combine to form atoms, the number of electrons and protons is always equal. This makes atoms stable because they are electrically neutral.

Neutrons are a little heavier than protons, but for practical purposes scientists say they weigh the same, which is 1.00 atomic mass unit or 1.00 amu.

Electrons are very small and light. It takes about 1,840 electrons to equal the mass of one proton or one neutron.

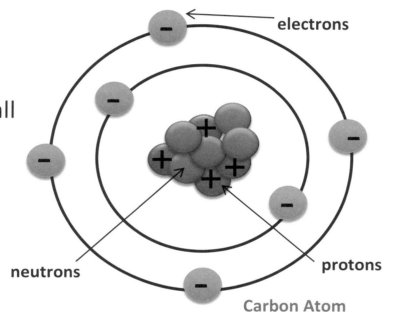

electrons

neutrons

protons

Carbon Atom

When you are finding the mass of an atom you are really only talking about the weight of the protons and neutrons because the electrons are basically weightless.

No matter the small size of an electron, it has a big negative electrical charge. It is so big it equals the proton's positive charge. This brings the atom into perfect electrical balance (electrically neutral again).

◆Simple Chemistry

Remember, the electrons and the protons in the atom are always equal. It is the number of neutrons that vary.

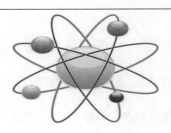

Model	Description
e / p / No neutrons / H	**Hydrogen Atom** • Smallest of all elements • 1.00 amu
e / pp / e / No neutrons / He	*Hypothetical* Helium Atom • Second lightest of all elements (see Stewart, chapter 3 for more information) • 2.00 amu
e / pp / nn / e / Two neutrons / He	Typical Helium Atom • True second lightest of all elements • 4.00 amu
e / pn / One neutron / H isotope*	Deuterium Atom • Heavy Hydrogen • 2.00 amu
e / p / nn / Two neutrons / H isotope*	Tritium Atom • Heavy Hydrogen • 3.00 amu

*An isotope is a difference of an element, in this case it is the number of neutrons in the nucleus.

You can see a pattern. As neutrons and protons are added to an element the atomic mass unit gets bigger!

◆Is Electricity in Every Chemical Process?

Yes, electricity is in every chemical process because in a strict sense chemistry is considered the study of *electrical exchanges between atoms involving only their shells of electrons and is not directly concerned with activities involving the nucleus.* This means that the activities involving the nucleus are the concern of physics, not chemistry.

The areas considered a *'chemical reaction'* have to do with sharing, borrowing, loaning, stealing, or giving up electrons between atoms. These activities of electrons orbiting in atoms are how compounds are formed and how they can be broken up.

When compounds break-up, for instance when an electrical current passes through water, the elements that make water return back to separate atoms of hydrogen and oxygen.

The Father of Chemistry, Antoine Laurent Lavoisier (1743-1794) stated, **"Nothing is lost, nothing is created. Everything is transformed**."

Antoine Laurent Lavoisier
is said to be
The Father of Chemistry

◆God's Plan for Creation in a Table

God created 92 natural elements and they all break down to different combinations of electrons, protons, and neutrons. It only takes two of these three building blocks to create hydrogen, but it takes all three to build the rest of the elements.

Hydrogen (H) atoms are the most numerous atoms of the universe and the lightest at *1.00 amu*. The heaviest naturally occurring element is Uranium (U) at 238.0 amu.

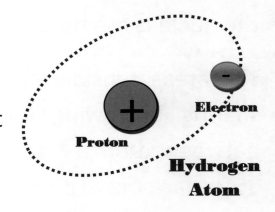

The Periodic Table lists the elements in order of their atomic numbers, 1 to 118; which is actually a listing by atomic weight. It is called periodic because the chemical properties repeat themselves as you go down the table.

The Periodic Table is constructed in 32 columns. The Lanthanides and Actinides' 14 columns are moved to the bottom so it will fit on one page.

Each column 'family' contains elements that have similar chemical characteristics.

◆The Periodic Table of Elements

The elements that have common characteristics can be considered families: metals, non-metals, and transitional elements.

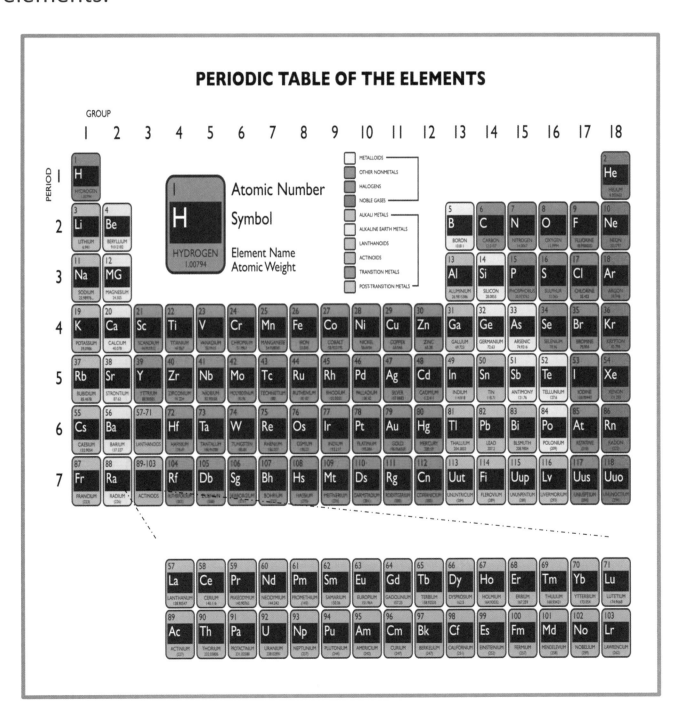

♦Who Discovered the Periodic Table?

The Russian scientist *Dmitri Ivanovitch Mendeleev* published his discovery of the Periodic Table in 1869. The interesting thing is that even though not all of the elements had been discovered yet, he knew where the remaining elements should be placed, so he left open spaces.

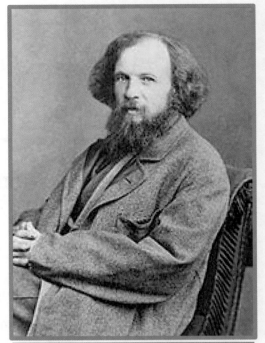

Dmitri Ivanovitch Mendeleev
(1884-1907)

Looking at the rows (periods) of the Periodic Table on page 23 you can see that the first period has only two elements (H and He). The second period contains eight elements (Li, Be, B, C, N, O, F, and Ne). The third period has eight elements (Na, Mg, Al, Si, P, S, Cl, and Ar). The fourth and fifth periods have 18 members, while the final sixth and seventh periods have 32 members each.

If you know how one element in a column behaves, you will know something about how every other element in that column behaves. They are family members and act alike.

◆How Do the Elements Act in the Body?

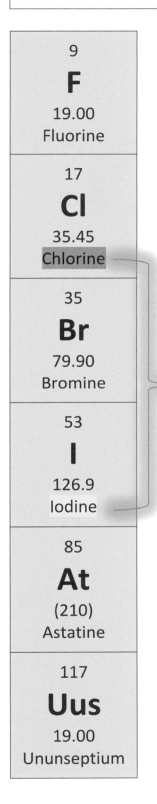

9	**F**
19.00	Fluorine
17	**Cl**
35.45	Chlorine
35	**Br**
79.90	Bromine
53	**I**
126.9	Iodine
85	**At**
(210)	Astatine
117	**Uus**
19.00	Ununseptium

All the elements in one column are family members. They are cousins that can change places with one another and this may not be a good thing for your body!

Iodine (I) is an element that is required for proper thyroid function. Notice that Chlorine (Cl) is a cousin of Iodine (I).

Many municipal water companies add chlorine to the city's water system to kill disease-causing bacteria; however, that means it is also in the water you drink. Chlorine is in the same column as iodine and can displace the iodine that is essential to your thyroid function.

The chlorine does not function in the body to support your thyroid so potentially the body could begin having thyroid related diseases: hyper or hypo-thyroidism.

◆Fragrance and Molecular Weight?

The atomic weight (atomic mass units or amu) of an element is simply the sum of the number of protons and neutrons in the nucleus of an atom.

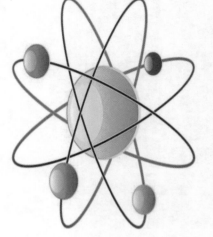

Molecular weight is important because it affects the way chemical compounds in essential oils behave: volatility, viscosity, and biological half-life.

- **Volatility**: is how fast oil evaporates. Small molecules will evaporate faster than large molecules.

- **Viscosity**: is the thickness of a liquid. Water is thin and runny, but honey is thicker and more viscous.

- **Biological half-life**: is the amount of time that it takes fifty percent of an oil to keep its aroma or maintain its action in the body.

The larger the molecule, the longer an applied oil will keep its aroma, therapeutic action, and the time it takes to be eliminated or metabolized.

◆The CHOSN Ones

Of the 92 natural elements on the Periodic Table, you only need to understand five of the elements as they relate to essential oils. Dr. Stewart calls these the "CHOSN Ones" because they were chosen by God from which to build life in its' billions of forms.

Carbon C_6

Hydrogen H_1

Oxygen O_8

Sulfur S_{16}

Nitrogen N_7

↖ amu

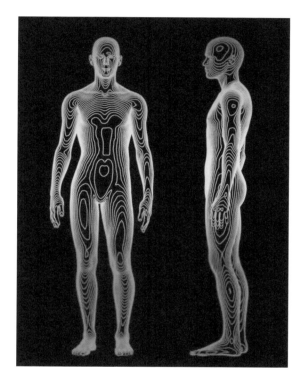

There is a considerable difference in size and weight (amu) between the CHOSN elements!

96 percent of our body is made-up of carbon, hydrogen, oxygen, and nitrogen. Sulfur and other trace elements make up the last four percent.

♦Atomic Models of CHOSN Elements

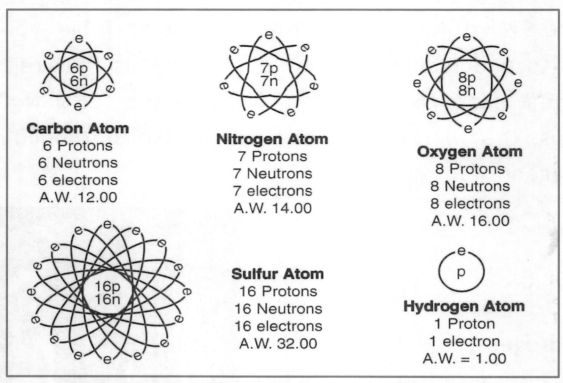

Carbon Atom
6 Protons
6 Neutrons
6 electrons
A.W. 12.00

Nitrogen Atom
7 Protons
7 Neutrons
7 electrons
A.W. 14.00

Oxygen Atom
8 Protons
8 Neutrons
8 electrons
A.W. 16.00

Sulfur Atom
16 Protons
16 Neutrons
16 electrons
A.W. 32.00

Hydrogen Atom
1 Proton
1 electron
A.W. = 1.00

Models from <u>Chemistry of Essential Oils Made Simple</u> (Stewart, 2005, p. 122)

The models above are vastly different in the way they look and in their molecular weight.

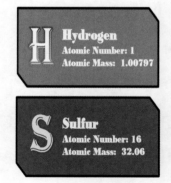

- *Hydrogen* has one proton and no neutrons and weighs in at 1.00 amu.

  H **Hydrogen**
  Atomic Number: 1
  Atomic Mass: 1.00797

- *Sulfur* has 16 protons and 16 neutrons with a weight of 32.00 amu.

  S **Sulfur**
  Atomic Number: 16
  Atomic Mass: 32.06

The **CHOSN** elements appear in the top three levels of the periodic table, are all non-metals, and do not conduct electricity.

♦What is a Valence?

Elements are like people: they like to have friends! Some elements like to have a lot of friends and others only want to have one best friend. This desire for friendship is called "valence."

The valence is due to the element's atoms and the electrons in the outer shells.

Carbon	(C)	4
Hydrogen	(H)	1
Oxygen	(O)	2
Sulfur	(S)	2
Nitrogen	(N)	3

Notice how both Oxygen and Sulfur have a valence of two. Remember how they are in the same column in the periodic table? All family members in each column of the periodic table have the same valence.

Look at the valences and you can see that Carbon is the party kid of the bunch! She likes to have four friends everywhere she goes.

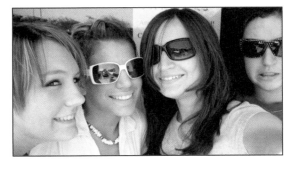

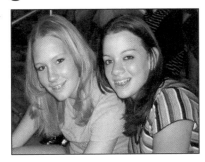

Hydrogen on the other hand likes to just have one best friend with her wherever she goes because she has a valence of one.

♦Cartoon Chemistry

Cartoons are a fun way to learn organic chemistry. Each **CHOSN** One's valence is represented using a cartoon character with a hand or hands to show how many friends it needs to be complete.

Hydrogen: H—✋

> A hydrogen atom with a valence of one is looking for one best friend.

Oxygen: ✋—O—✋   Sulfur: ✋—S—✋

> Oxygen and sulfur are cousins and are both looking for two friends.

Nitrogen: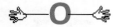

> Nitrogen is a different configuration and is looking for three people to party with.

Carbon: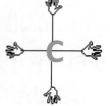

> Carbon is the most social of all the CHOSN ones and is looking for a large party of four to satisfy its need for group fun.

(See David Stewart's <u>The Chemistry of Essential Oils Made Simple</u> (2005) chapter four pgs. 121-141)

♦From Cartoons to Organic Chemistry

Let's imagine there is one oxygen floating and it is looking for two friends. He finds two separate hydrogen atoms and they all grasp hands:

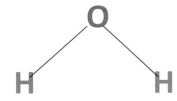

Now you have a satisfied and happy group of friends:
- Oxygen is happy because he has both hands held.
- The hydrogens are happy because they each have one hand held.

What do you have when you put one oxygen with two hydrogens? H_2O!

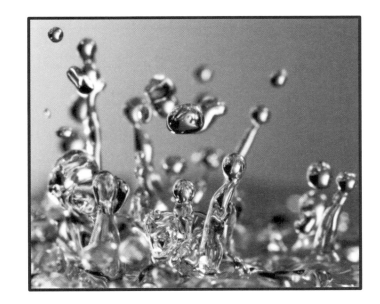

You now have the chemical formula of water! All that from simple cartoons. Well done!

♦Knowledge of Cartoons to Learn More

Remember that sulfur and oxygen are cousins? Let's use the same chemical formula, but switch out the cousins. H_2S!

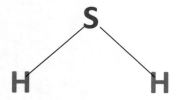

This is the chemical formula for Hydrogen Sulfide "rotten egg gas". In other words H_2**Stinky**!

Carbon is the biggest collector of friends in our **CHOSN** group. Let's see how his valences work. He likes to have four friends. We will give him a hydrogen to hold onto for each of his hands. That gives us the chemical formula of CH_4.

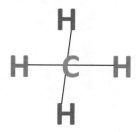

This is a molecule of methane gas. It has the odor of rotting leaves. Another stinky one!

♦Expanding on Valences

Now that you understand the concept of valences you know that each atom must be satisfied to create a complete molecule. However, not all molecules are created in the same way.

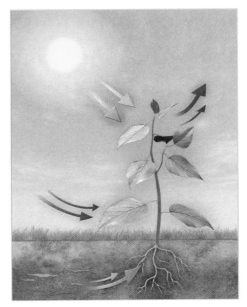

When we inhale fresh oxygen (O_2) we exhale carbon dioxide (CO_2) which is what plants breathe in to create oxygen. It is a wonderful cycle because we depend on each other to sustain life.

Carbon dioxide is a satisfied molecule

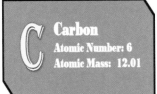

Carbon
Atomic Number: 6
Atomic Mass: 12.01

because all of its bonds are satisfied, but in a different way. It is happy because of a 'double-bond'.

O   C   O

Unlike the bonds in water where it looks more like the sides of a triangle, these bonds run straight from one pair to the other satisfying each other's need for company.

◆Organic Chemistry

When you hear the word 'organic' what do you think of?

Most people say things like: healthy, no pesticides, good for the body, or naturally grown. That may have been true in the past, but a strict definition is simply *"pertaining to a class of chemical compounds that formerly comprised only those existing in or derived from plants or animals, but that now includes all other compounds of carbon."* (dictionary.com)

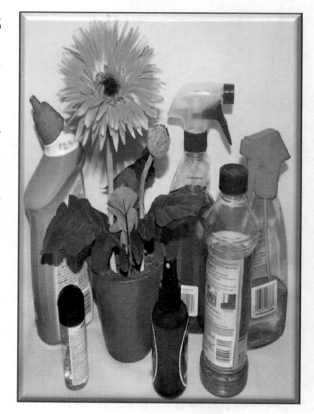

Every living thing on earth is made of carbon compounds. Scientists can also make carbon compounds in a lab. These lab-made compounds are not natural compounds, but because they contain carbon...they can be labeled organic.

Products like chemical bug sprays, gasoline, and motor oil can be called organic too, but they are poisonous to the human body. Read labels carefully when buying something that states it is 'organic'.

♦When Does Natural Mean Natural?

The United States Federal Government allows people to use the word 'natural' on a product label **IF** the compounds that make up the product **'could'** be produced in nature.

That means that even if the product was made in a lab or factory using chemicals, but could have been made of natural products, it can be labeled 'natural'.

Manufacturers do this because they don't think that it matters whether a product was made in nature or a lab.

Nature Made	Factory Made

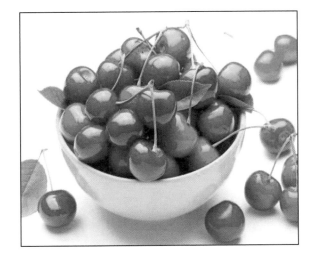

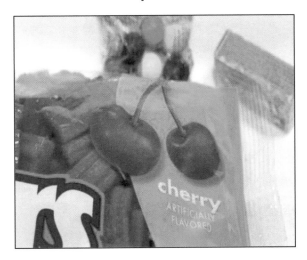

Natural Cherries

Cherry flavor created by God

Cherry Flavored Candy

Cherry flavor created by man with chemicals to fake God's creation

Examples: Sugar, Corn Syrup, High Fructose Corn Syrup, Citric Acid, Artificial Flavor, Colors (Red 40, Blue 1)

♦Oils that Heal and Those that Don't

Natural therapeutic grade essential oils enter the body with the purpose of bringing health to sick or confused organs, to resolve emotional issues stored in the body, and provide balanced organization to our body's systems.

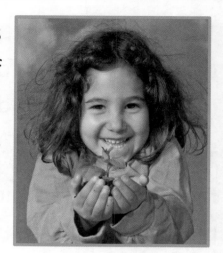

Dr. Stewart stated, "This organizing power is what the term organic originally meant." Order and health are harmonious in the body. Disorder and sickness are disharmonious in the body and cause disease. Only true therapeutic grade essential oils bring harmony to the body.

Natural Therapeutic Grade
(unadulterated)

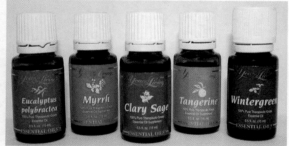

Amber bottles, labels show full ingredients, include botanical name, and have healing power

Synthetic Grade
(food or perfume)

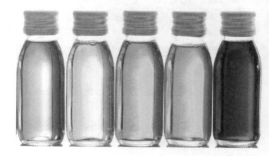

Clear bottles, labels do not show full ingredients or botanical name, and lack healing power

♦What is a Hydrocarbon?

A hydrocarbon is a simple molecule containing only hydrogen and carbon, so we call them *'hydrocarbons'*.

hydro + carbon = hydrocarbon

Methane gas CH_4 is the simplest hydrocarbon.

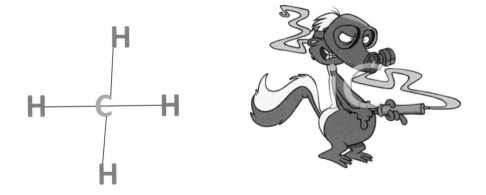

Remember:

Carbon's valence is 4 and hydrogen's valence is 1.

The simplest possible hydrocarbon would be to begin with one carbon and let it make friends with as many hydrogen atoms as it chooses. Then link two or more carbons with more hydrogens to make long chains.

◆Methane is a Hydrocarbon

Methane gas is part of the Alkane family.

The Alkane family starts out small with methane gas.

It has one **Carbon atom and four Hydrogen atoms which equals** CH_4.

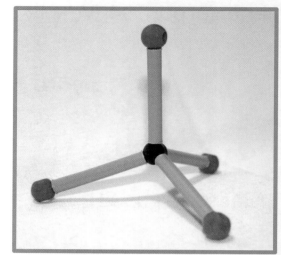

This family does not stay small, in fact, it grows very large. This growth actually happens in a very easy to follow mathematical pattern C_nH_{2n+2}.

Note: *Hydrocarbons should <u>not</u> be confused with carbohydrates.*

Carbohydrate compounds are created from water molecules and carbon atoms and are building blocks of bread, pasta, potatoes, grains, and sugar.

Hydrate = water or H_2O.

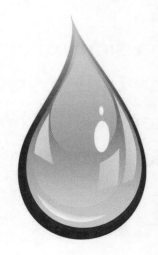

◆Alkane Family Formula

The Alkane family is easy to learn because it has a pattern. The alkane pattern has a mathematical formula that looks like this: C_nH_{2n+2}

Take the number of carbons which are represented by 'n' and multiply it by 2, and then add 2.

CH_4	Methane	
C_2H_6	Ethane	
C_3H_8	Propane	
C_4H_{10}	Butane	
C_5H_{12}	Pentane	
C_6H_{14}	Hexane	
C_7H_{16}	Heptane	
C_8H_{18}	Octane	

(See <u>Chemistry of Essential Oils Made Simple</u> by Stewart, 2005, p. 148)

All of these compounds are *'Alkane Family'* members and hydrocarbons.

♦Would a Rose Smell as Sweet?

Rose oil contains the highest concentration of alkanes in an essential oil. It can contain up to 19% alkanes, but the average percentage is around 11%. By contrast, ginger has a much lower concentration at 1%. Except for trace amounts, alkanes are not found in the vast majority of essential oils.

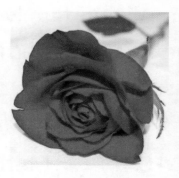

The oil of a rose petal contains at least ten different alkane molecules. These are heavy molecules and because of that weight they are less volatile. The size and weight of these molecules provide a longer lasting therapeutic action and staying power of the fragrance.

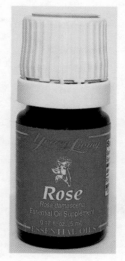

The 11-19% of alkanes might not seem like a lot at first, but consider that even 1% of any one ingredient in an oil is considered a major ingredient and you can see that alkanes play a huge part of why a rose is a rose. If you have ever felt a rose petal's waxy texture, you have felt an alkane.

Fun Fact: It takes 5000 pounds of rose petals to make 1 pound of rose oil.

♦What is a Radical?

Dr. Stewart defines radicals as "*Incomplete molecules looking for something to which to attach themselves in order to satisfy their unfulfilled appetites.*" (pg. 153).

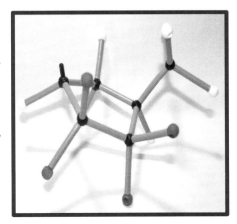

This means that one of the hands of the molecule is not holding onto a friend and so she goes in search of a friend to hold hands with.

Methyl is one of those radicals. Anytime you read a compound with "methyl" in its name, it contains a methyl radical in the molecule. Two very common ones in essential oils are:

> **Methyl salicylate**: *a disinfectant antiseptic found in wintergreen oil.*
>
> **Methyl chavicol**: strongly antispasmodic and found in **basil oil**.

♦What is Methyl's Attraction?

In the world of essential oils Methyl must be a very good friend because she has been invited to be a part of hundreds of thousands of compounds. When you see 'methyl' in a compound think to yourself, "Oh, it has one carbon." An example of how a radical occurs is below:

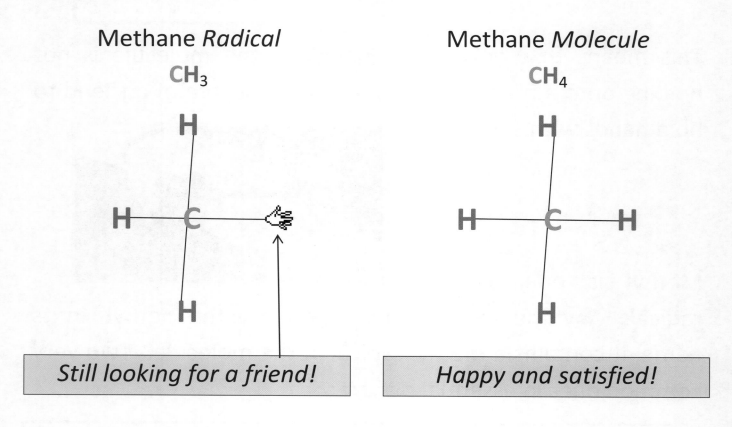

Methane *Radical*

CH_3

Methane *Molecule*

CH_4

Still looking for a friend!

Happy and satisfied!

In this example you have a happy methane molecule, but then something happens and one of the hydrogens gets knocked off. Then Methyl Radical goes looking for a friend to grab onto. Sometimes there may even be two hydrogen molecules missing, but is it still called a methyl.

◆The Radical Sisters

Methyl is not the only radical. She has a whole group of sisters that act just like her! These sisters are partial molecules:

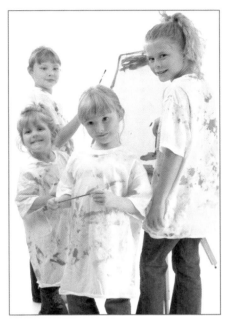

- Have their hands out looking for a friend to grab on to
- Incomplete and unbalanced
- All very popular and asked to join many compounds

The Methane radical on the previous page shows one carbon attached to three hydrogen and one searching hand out.

The second radical sister looks very much like her sister, but larger. She has two carbons attached to five hydrogens and one hand out searching for a friend. This pattern of adding carbons and hydrogens continues with the other sisters: Propyl and Butyl.

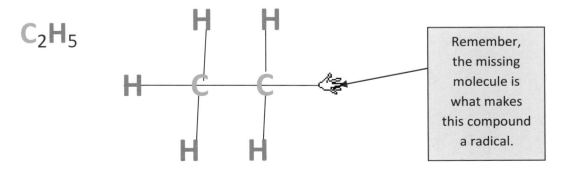

C_2H_5

Remember, the missing molecule is what makes this compound a radical.

◆Oxygenated Hydrocarbons

Dr. Stewart defines the chemistry of essential oils as:

"Simple hydrocarbons, oxygenated hydrocarbons, and their isomers."

This is an important step in our learning about chemistry because we are now moving away from compounds with two elements to compounds with three elements. They are called oxygenated hydrocarbons.

An oxygenated hydrocarbon is a compound. It is considered a compound because it has two or more different chemical elements.

Oxygenated hydrocarbons contain the elements of hydrogen, carbon, and oxygen.

Carbon + **Hydrogen** = **Hydrocarbon**

Hydrocarbon + **Oxygen** = <u>**Oxygenated Hydrocarbon**</u>

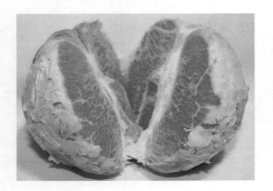

Limonene, g-terpinene, myrcene and a-pinene are several abundant hydrocarbons in the essential oil of tangerine.

♦From Alkanes to Alcohols

We have already learned about the Alkane family with its pattern and mathematical formulas. Introducing an oxygen atom it transforms alkanes to alcohols which produces new family members known as:

methanol, *ethanol*, **propanol**, *and* **butanol**.

They now have different physical and chemical properties.

When a molecule such as *Ethane* becomes oxygenated it converts to an alcohol known as *Ethanol*.

Ethane C_2H_6

            4 carbon atoms

            6 hydrogen atoms

Ethanol C_2H_6O

            4 carbon atoms

            6 hydrogen atoms

            1 oxygen atom

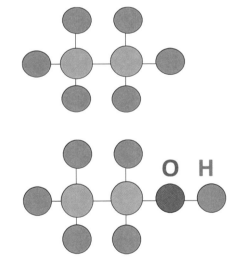

In this instance the Alkane family become oxygenated by a hydroxyl radical (**OH**) and turns into an alcohol. Their names no longer end in –ane, they now end in –ol.

♦From Alkanes to Alcohols Continued

In the visuals below you can see that when a member of the Alkane family is oxygenated by adding an OH to one end, it goes from being a flammable gas to an alcoholic liquid.

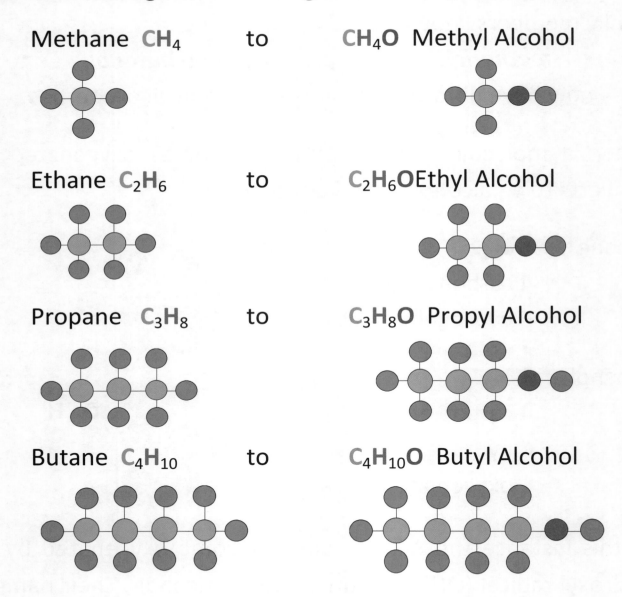

Methane **CH₄** to **CH₄O** Methyl Alcohol

Ethane **C₂H₆** to **C₂H₆O** Ethyl Alcohol

Propane **C₃H₈** to **C₃H₈O** Propyl Alcohol

Butane **C₄H₁₀** to **C₄H₁₀O** Butyl Alcohol

Most perfumes containing essential oils contain over 90% ethyl alcohol.

◆Alcohols and Essential Oils

There are many kinds of alcohols in essential oils.

Some people express a concern that using too many essential oils at one time can make you drunk.

Don't worry.

The only alcohol that makes you drunk

Is ethyl alcohol C_2H_6O

which is *not* found in essential oils.

In chemistry, any hydrocarbon with an **OH** attached is an alcohol by definition.

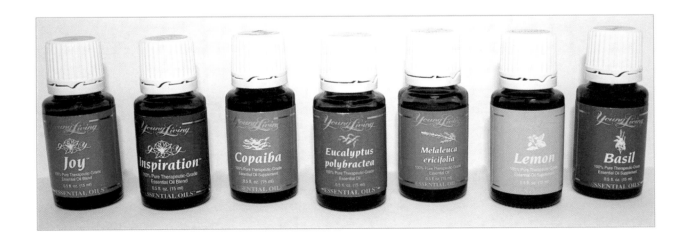

◆Isomers

We know that Dr. Stewart stated, *"The chemistry of essential oils consists of simple hydrocarbons, oxygenated hydrocarbons, and their isomers"*. We now need to learn about what isomers are.

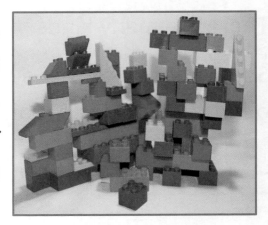

The Greek name **isomers** simply means "**same parts**":

    Isos = equal or the same

    Meros = parts

Isomers have the same building blocks, but they have been created in different formations or structures.

Essentially, isomers are re-arrangements of atoms to create compounds with the same chemical formula.

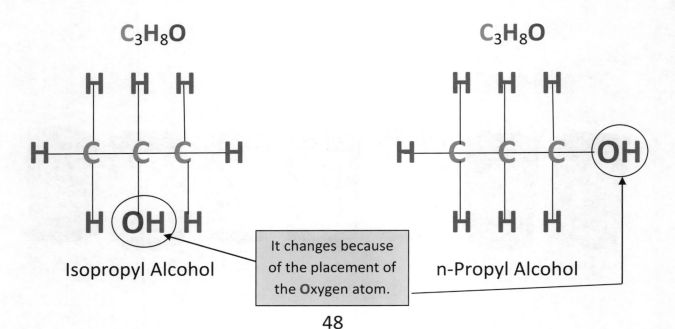

C_3H_8O — Isopropyl Alcohol

C_3H_8O — n-Propyl Alcohol

It changes because of the placement of the **O**xygen atom.

48

◆What do Legos have to do with Isomers?

Using Legos® helps us to imagine all the different possibilities for molecular formulas created by isomers.

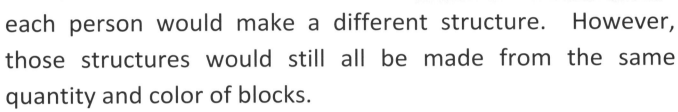

If you give several people 8 red, 3 blue , and 5 yellow Legos each person would make a different structure. However, those structures would still all be made from the same quantity and color of blocks.

A formula for those building blocks would look like this:

$$R_8B_3Y_5$$

If you gave 100 people the same color and quantity of Legos there are numerous possibilities of structures to be created. If computed, the number would come out to **20,922,789,888,000.** That is over 20-trillion possibilities!

These 20-trillion possibilities are all *'isomers'* of the same chemical formula. Dr. Stewart likes to say that *"Atoms are God's Legos"* and they are the building blocks of every molecule on earth, including essential oils.

♦A Puzzling Compound

In 1825, a new compound called Benzene was discovered. It was a puzzling compound for scientists because they knew that its formula was C_6H_6, but they could not figure out how to draw its structure with the proper valences.

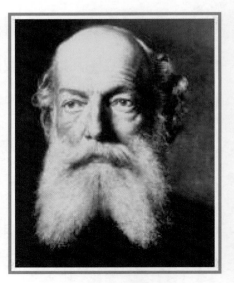

Friedrich August Kekulé
German Chemist
1829–1896

The problem was at that time they did not know how six hydrogen atoms (H_6) would be able to fulfill the appetites of six carbon atoms (C_6) and form a stable compound. It just did not add up.

Then along came Friedrich August Kekulé, a German chemist. He was one of the first to realize that carbon atoms like to form chains. These chains attract other elements such as:

Hydrogen, Oxygen, Sulfur, and Nitrogen.

Then they can become three-dimensional entities.

Kekulé had a special talent and interest in visualizing these structures and was a pioneer in the field of the structural architecture of chemistry. He had a dream...

50

◆Kekulé's Dancing Snakes

One evening in 1866 Kekulé was sitting in front of his fireplace after a long day trying to figure out the C_6H_6 puzzle. He was tired and dozed-off. During this time he had a dream that there were atoms dancing in front of his eyes. These atoms formed chains and these chains morphed into dancing snakes.

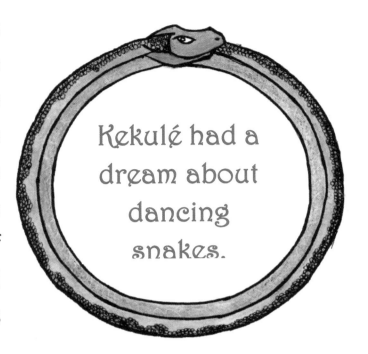

Kekulé had a dream about dancing snakes.

He was mesmerized as he watched one snake twist and turn and finally wrapped around and grabbed its tail in its own mouth. Just then Kekulé's eyes flew open and he knew exactly what the structure of C_6H_6 should look like! It is in a ring!!

This dream illustrated for Kekulé that carbon would not only form chains, but also rings. This solved the puzzle that had been haunting scientists for 41 years.

Kekulé won a Nobel Prize for his work, and in 2005 the United States Postal Service issued a stamp in his honor.

♦Aromatic Rings

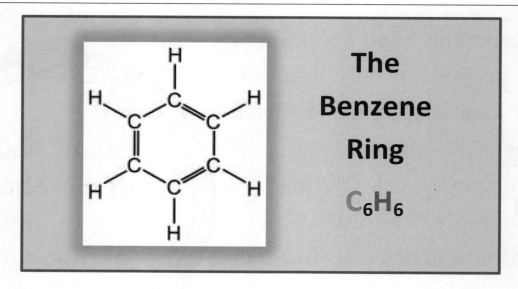

The Benzene Ring

C_6H_6

Benzene or carbon rings play major roles in *every* essential oil, which is why they are called "**aromatic rings**" by chemists.

Remember back on page 34 when we learned about double bonds? Such as: O====C====O or CO_2?

The bonds in Benzene rings are double bonds, but they alternate from single to double. That means that two arms of a carbon atom are holding onto the same atom, which just happens to be another carbon.

This ring occurs so frequently as part of larger molecules, scientists had to come-up with an easy way to represent it without all those **H**'s and **C**'s being written out. This is called a shorthand formula.

♦Shorthand for Aromatic Rings

Shorthand formulas omit the symbols for hydrogen and carbon altogether. Instead it is drawn as a simple hexagon with alternating double bonds.

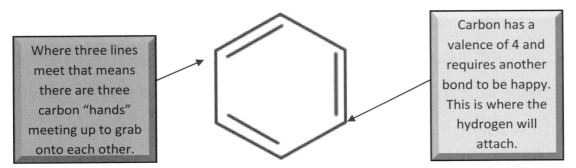

Where three lines meet that means there are three carbon "hands" meeting up to grab onto each other.

Carbon has a valence of 4 and requires another bond to be happy. This is where the hydrogen will attach.

Visualize a **C** (carbon) atom at each junction above. From each of the junctions there will be an **H** (hydrogen) atom attached. Why does each junction need a hydrogen to be happy?

Remember that carbons have a valence of four and hydrogen has a valence of one. Each junction above has three carbons meeting and the attached hydrogen completes the valence requirement. This makes everyone happy and satisfied. It is a stable compound.

Using this shorthand method a chemical formula for a hydrocarbon can be figured out even if the **C**'s and **H**'s are not drawn out.

⬥Aromatic Rings into Quantum Physics

The Benzene ring has a very dynamic personality. When six carbons join with six hydrogens their electrons are not best friends with any one atom. They move around all over the ring and hang out with everyone. They are called "delocalized" electrons which means they are not confined to orbit a single atom. They are still in the molecule, but just have a much larger neighborhood in which to play, move, and explore.

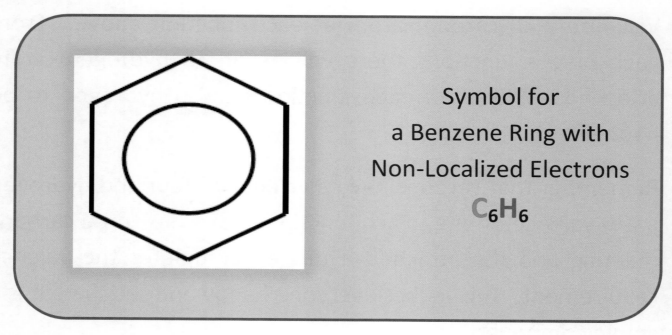

Symbol for
a Benzene Ring with
Non-Localized Electrons
C_6H_6

Due to all this moving around in a large neighborhood scientists don't actually know where the double bonds occur because the bonds are not stationary. So, scientists created another short hand version for the benzene ring to represent all this movement.

⬥Benzene Rings and Electromagnetic Frequencies

Just like children running around a neighborhood generate a lot of energy, these atoms running around their ring have generated megahertz frequencies (millions of time per second). These resonance generating atoms give therapeutic grade essential oils their frequencies. The electrons are dashing around the molecules instead of being tied to just one friendly atom. We call this "resonance energy" of the molecule.

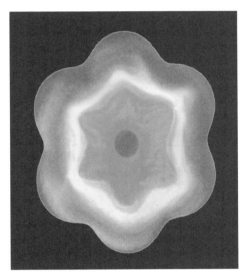

This picture shows an aromatic benzene ring as a nebulous hexagon of electromagnetic frequencies and intensities present in the molecule.

A pulsating atom with non-localized electrons is no longer considered matter because it has been transformed into a waveform—a bundle of energy.

Dr. Stewart stated, "*The wavelike nature of benzene and other functional groups with aromatic rings leads directly into relativity and quantum physics which takes us to a hybrid field of science called nuclear chemistry and leads to consciousness itself, including both our consciousness and that of God (p. 177).*"

Note: See Part III of <u>Chemistry of Essential Oils Made Easy</u> for more details.

♦Frequencies and Essential Oils

A German physicist Heinrich Rudolph Hertz discovered electro-magnetic radiation known as radio waves in 1888. In his honor, the electromagnetic frequencies are measured in "Hertz" with an abbreviation of "hz".

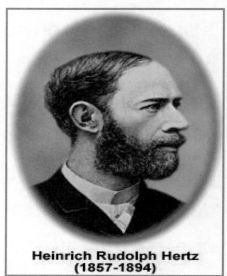

Heinrich Rudolph Hertz (1857-1894)

Within every molecule of essential oils there is a whole spectrum of vibrational frequencies. The larger the molecule the more complex the spectrum of frequency gets and the greater the range.

The double bonds in essential oil molecules vibrate so quickly that they have to be measured in mega-megahertz (MMhz).

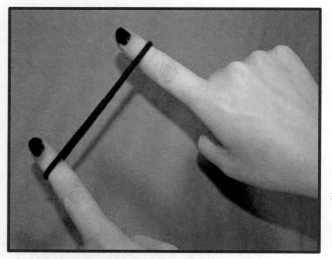

This can be visualized by imagining rubber-bands stretched between pairs of atoms. Each time the band moves it creates a vibration and then a sound. Each bond creates a different vibration and therefore a different sound. It is this vibration that gives essential oils their frequency.

♦Frequencies and Coherence

As you can imagine, there are millions of different bonds in one drop of essential oil and each of these bonds are vibrating at a different frequency. It seems like the results would give rise to mass chaos! However, it does not. Instead they all function together like a symphony orchestra tuned in harmonious mathematical precision.

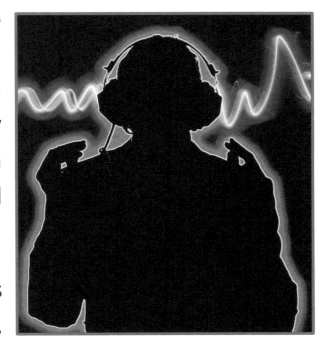

Dr. Stewart refers to this precisional vibration as, "**Natural compounds being blended by God to create a healing oil**". The molecules are imbued with God's word and respond to one another and adjust their frequencies into the coherence of a finely tuned instrument.

The molecules of therapeutic grade essential oils are functional families that form coherent and harmonious groups, without dissonance or disharmony, allowing healing vibrations to enter our bodies.

♦The Significance of Frequency

Essential oils resonate with your bodily tissues when they are inhaled, swallowed, or applied to the skin. The different frequencies in essential oils increase the body's own natural electromagnetic vibrations and can produce healing through elevating the body to its proper frequency.

If the body's fundamental frequencies fall below a certain level, the body may catch a cold or the flu. If they drop lower, the body can be susceptible to serious diseases. The table below provides the fundamental frequencies of people, food, herbs, and essential oils.

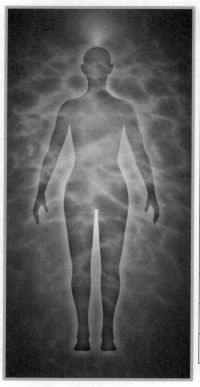

Frequencies of People and Things	Megahertz
Healthy Human Brain	71-90
Healthy Human Body	62-68
Human Body with Cold Symptoms	58
Human Body with Flu Symptoms	57
Human Body with Cancer	42
Human Body beginning to die	25
Processed or Canned Foods	0
Fresh Produce	10-15
Dry Herbs	12-22
Fresh Herbs	20-27
Therapeutic Grade Essential Oils	52-320

(See Chemistry of Essential Oils Made Simple by Stewart, p. 182)

♦The Fundamental Frequencies

The fundamental frequencies of the body respond to and fluctuate because of the types of food we eat. The table on the previous page shows that canned food registers at a zero frequency, but fresh produce registers between 10-15 mhz. Do you know which one would be better for the body?

Just like the difference in canned and fresh food, the body's frequencies respond to our thoughts: negative or positive, dissonant or peaceful.

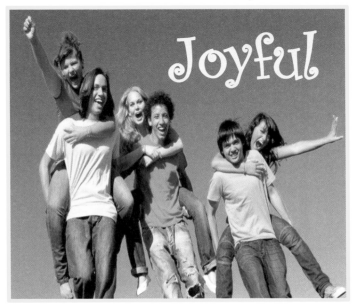

Our emotions also play a part in the body's electromagnetic frequency and can keep us healthy or put us at risk to sickness. Love, faith, calmness, and joy all raise our body's frequencies while emotions such as hate, envy, fear, and pride can lower our body's frequencies.

Essential oils help 'sick organs' of the body come back into frequency by getting into the body, finding the organ that has a similar 'sound' and then reminding it to vibrate at its proper frequency.

♦Benzene Rings Get Oxygenated

There are many active parts of essential oils, but some of the most active compounds are called "phenols" or "phenolics". **Phenolics** contain a benzene ring with a hydroxyl radical attached. The formula is C_6H_6O.

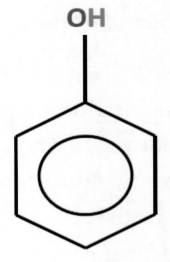

Phenols end in –*ol* and we previously learned all compounds that end in –ol are alcohols; therefore, phenols are alcohols. However, these are special compounds with very different properties from other alcohols.

Phenols are strong substances and are found in small concentrations in essential oils such as cinnamon and cassia. However, they play a large part in many oils like oregano and thyme. When phenols play with other molecules it is called a 'functional group'.

A functional group is a complete molecule willing to join with others. A phenol is one such molecule because it is built on a benzene ring and the compounds that contain a phenol functional group are called phenolics.

♦Phenolics to Functional Groups

Phenolic oils cleanse receptor sites on cells and have many healing benefits. They may boost the immune system, detoxify the body, and make environments unfriendly to bacteria. Oils containing Phenols are:

Oil Name	Percentage	Bottle Label
Wintergreen	97%	
Clove	77%	
Basil	76%	
Rose	3%	
Myrrh	1%	

Some oils containing phenols are strong and can irritate the skin. Dilute these oils with V6 oil or other organic vegetable oil as needed.

◆Phenylpropanoids

Phenylpropanoids are another critical molecule in therapeutic grade essential oils. They are created when a *'propyl radical'* and a *'phenol molecule'* hook-up and become friends.

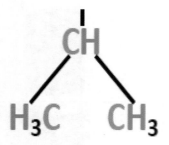

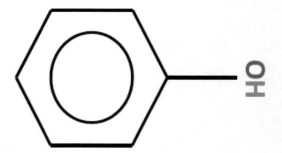

Propyl Radical with a three-carbon chain is an incomplete molecule so it goes looking for someone to grab onto.

Phenol is a happy compound because all of its valences are satisfied, but it is also very social. When it sees an unsatisfied propyl radical it wants to make friends.

When a phenol compound locates a propyl radical they form together to make a phenylpropanoid. Phenylpropanoids are compounds that give essential oils the ability to cleanse the receptor sites of cells and allow the process of healing at the cellular level to begin. They also assist our bodies in maintaining wellness on a daily basis.

♦Reading Structural Formulas

Diagramming the simplest phenylpropanoid provides an easy way to learn how to read structural formulas of essential oils. The compound below is called 'p-cuminol' or 'australol'. It can be found in the essential oils of eucalyptus and cumin. Each of the diagrams below are for the same formula: C_9H_7O.

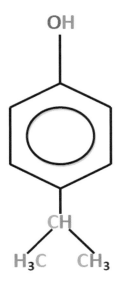

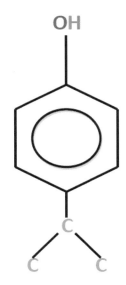

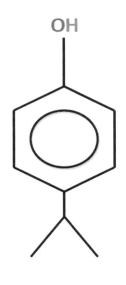

C_9H_7O	C_9H_7O	C_9H_7O
Explicit formula showing the three-carbon propyl chain CH_3CHCH_3	Explicit formula that omits the hydrogens, but with the knowledge that there will be hydrogens connecting each carbon	Shorthand formula that omits all notation with the knowledge that there is a carbon at each junction and hydrogens connecting to each carbon

♦Introduction to Biochemistry

Our bodies have a master DNA blue print inside each cell. There are about 100 trillion cells in the body and each of those cells have six gigabytes of memory.

That is more memory than if you hooked all the computers in the world together!

Our bodies are so perfectly created that each cell contains a master blue print of our whole body and appears holographically.

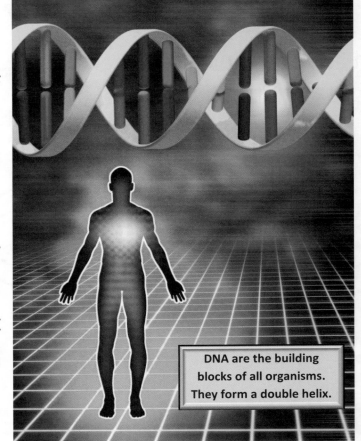

DNA are the building blocks of all organisms. They form a double helix.

If you cut a cell into pieces each piece would contain the same blueprint. This is why scientists have been able to clone a complete living animal from one cell because all the diversity of its organs and tissues can be generated from a single cell.

Aren't bodies and cells just fascinating?!

♦100 Trillion Cells as Employees

Let's consider your 100 trillion cells to be employees who work for you. You don't have to worry about organizing their function because they know what to do. They all have very specific jobs and can be illustrated in the following ways:

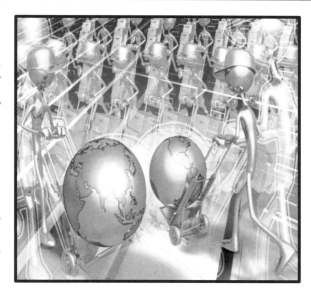

Nervous System	Endocrine System	Cyto-Kine System
"Text System" (sending simple messages)	**"Federal Express"** (sending complex messages)	**"Intercellular Messengers"** (as needed 24 hours a day)
• Messages sent by wire • Simple motor commands • Via simple electrical signal • Example: stepping on a rock, feeling pain, and jerking your foot up	• Use ligands to communicate through membranes • Talk to DNA • Read endocrine organs • Examples: digesting a pizza or soda pop, or fight off a cold or flu virus	• Millions of types • Involves every cell in the body as a source of ligands • Work globally throughout the body • Example: going red in the face over being embarrassed

Essential oil molecules support, enhance, and blend with all of these systems in ways that are physically, emotionally, and spiritually beneficial.

♦Alphabet Toting Hormonal Peptides

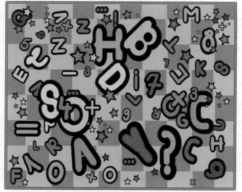

Peptides are chains of amino acids. They are fascinating because they form words and sentences that the body reads and understands.

When we eat the proper foods the body uses 20 essential amino acids. These 20 amino acids are like 20 individual letters in our body, a molecular alphabet so to speak. If you compare that to our 26 letter alphabet with all the words and sentences we can make, you can tell just how well this alphabet creates conversations within the cells. Basically, there is no limit on what it can say except that its phrases must be 100 characters or less to be small enough to pass through the cells in the body. Think of it like your body is sending a tweet!

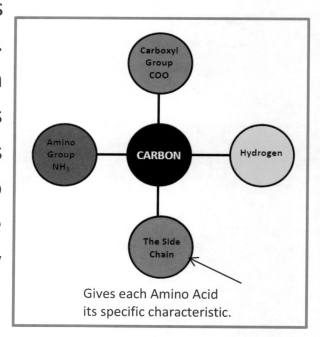

Gives each Amino Acid its specific characteristic.

Remember that for anything to get into our cells it has to be smaller than 500 amu.

♦Receiving of Hormones

I bet you are wondering how a hormone that wants to send a message to your heart gets to the correct location. There is an easy answer to a very complex process. It sings its way there!

On the surface of all cells are thousands of message readers called 'receptor sites'. These receptor sites are designed to accept only certain types of messages. This is important because you would not want a message sent to your heart to be intercepted and read by your liver. This would confuse your whole body!

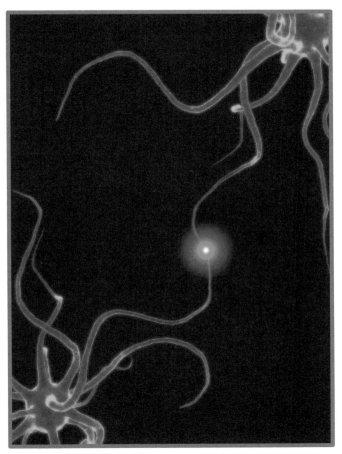

Picture of two cells communicating

When a hormone is released into the blood stream it sings a song and the correct receptor site will sing back to it so it knows where to go.

♦Ligands are the Messengers

The messengers that carry the information to cells and organs in our body are called 'ligands'.

In one sense, ligands are like keys that fit only certain receptor sites which are like little locks on the cells. To unlock the cell a ligand has to be the right shape or molecular structure to fit the cell or organ it is trying to get into.

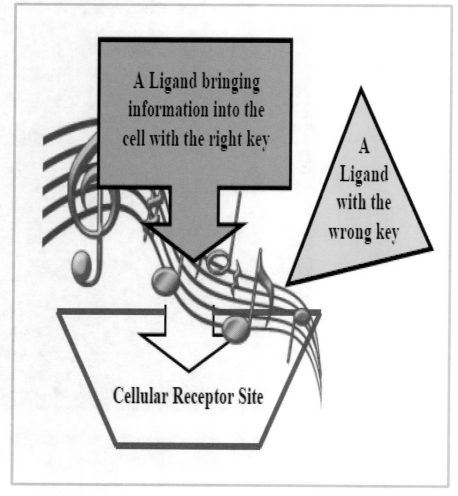

A Ligand bringing information into the cell with the right key

A Ligand with the wrong key

Cellular Receptor Site

The ligands of other shapes are rejected because their keys don't fit.

These ligand messengers know where to go in the body because each cell whistles a tune that the ligand can hear and follow to unlock the cell using the perfect key.

◆Cell Structures are Mini Cities

Imagine New York City with all of its buildings, streets, schools, churches, sewer plants, people, electrical lines, phone lines, water pipes, government offices, police and fire stations, etc.

Imagine shrinking it all down to fit on the head of a pin.

Now, imagine it even smaller and you still will not be able to get a perfect picture of the inner workings of one cell in our bodies. Human cells are so complicated that scientists have not been able to completely understand the biology of the inner workings of our cells.

♦Isomers: Right and Left "Chiral Pairs"

Remember that isomers are compounds of the same formula with a different structure. The compound below is called carvone $C_{10}H_{14}O$.

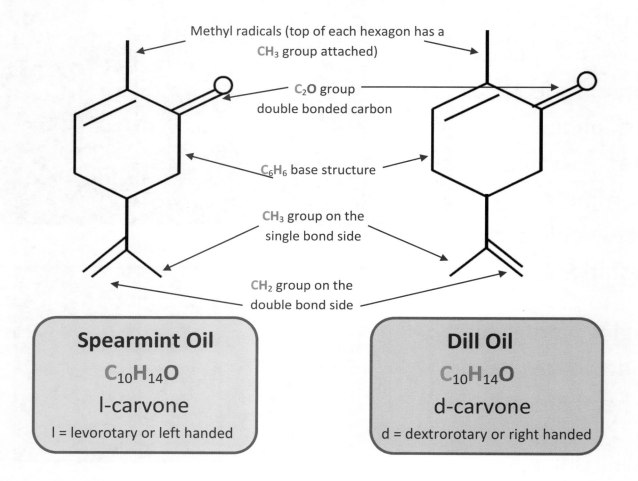

Methyl radicals (top of each hexagon has a CH_3 group attached)

C_2O group
double bonded carbon

C_6H_6 base structure

CH_3 group on the single bond side

CH_2 group on the double bond side

Spearmint Oil

$C_{10}H_{14}O$

l-carvone

l = levorotary or left handed

Dill Oil

$C_{10}H_{14}O$

d-carvone

d = dextrorotary or right handed

These two compounds are propanoids because a propyl radical is attached to the benzene ring. Notice that they do not have **OH** radicals attached to their hexagonal rings, and therefore are not considered phenylpropanoids.

♦The Nose Knows the Molecular Structure

These two $C_{10}H_{14}O$ compounds are almost exactly alike except for one small molecular difference, but that small difference can be picked up by our noses!

Isomers that come in left and right handed pairs are called 'chiral moelcules'. **Chiral** is greek for **hand**, such as **chiro**practors who adjust bodies with their hands.

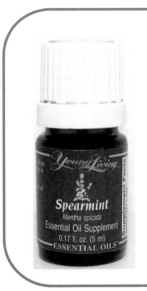

Spearmint Properties:
- ♦ Releases emotional blocks
- ♦ Weight loss
- ♦ Promotes a feeling of balance

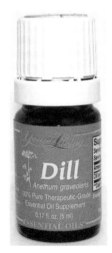

Dill Properties:
- ♦ Antibacterial
- ♦ Stimulant
- ♦ Reduces anxiety

It is amazing how the receptor sites in our noses can tell which way a propyl unit is turned on a tiny molecule, but it can. These two oils don't smell anything like each other, nor do they invoke the same emotional response.

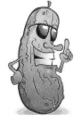

Imagine eating spearmint pickles or dill flavored gum? Most likely your taste buds would argue!

♦Keys that Open and Those that Don't

The carvone examples on the previous page illustrate how a slight difference in a molecular structure can be picked-up by our noses and stir up differences in our body, mind, and emotions.

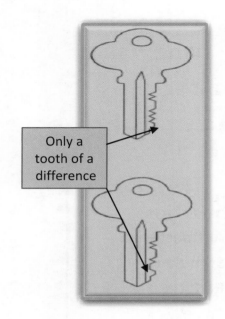

Only a tooth of a difference

To illustrate this point look at these two keys. They have both been cut from the same master key, but one turns on a fancy car and the other opens an old clunker.

These two keys will fit into the same locks, but they will not be able to open them. The tiniest difference in a key completely changes what it will or will not open.

It is the same concept we have with the two carvone molecules. One is right-handed and one is left-handed. Trying to get them into each other's receptor site is like trying to put a left hand glove onto your right hand...it just doesn't work.

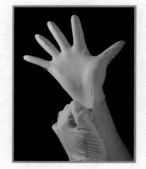

L-carvone sends messages to the cells in the pancreas while D-carvone sends messages to the gall bladder, intestines, and uterus.

♦Essential Oils: Biochemical Agents

Essential oils function in our bodies just like ligands. They get into the body and listen for a cell to sing a tune just like their own because that is the location they are needed and will be beneficial.

Essential oils can act just like hormones, vitamins, transmitters, enzymes, or antibiotics. They can be cleansing, immunizing, detoxifying, balancing, and mood elevating, all depending upon the receptor sites they open and what the body has stored there.

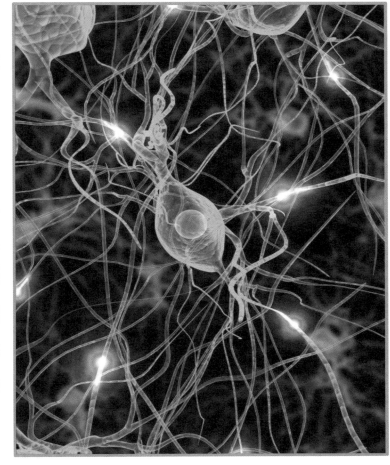

Essential oils have intelligence. They understand what parts of the body are carrying blocked feelings, diseases, toxins, and microbes. They go directly to that spot, open the lock, and walk right in to assist the body in healing itself. We don't have to do anything more than get them onto and into the body!

♦Similar Shapes, Different Fragrances

The nose knows! Grab a bottle of oregano and one of thyme and smell each oil. Your nose can tell the unique odors of each.

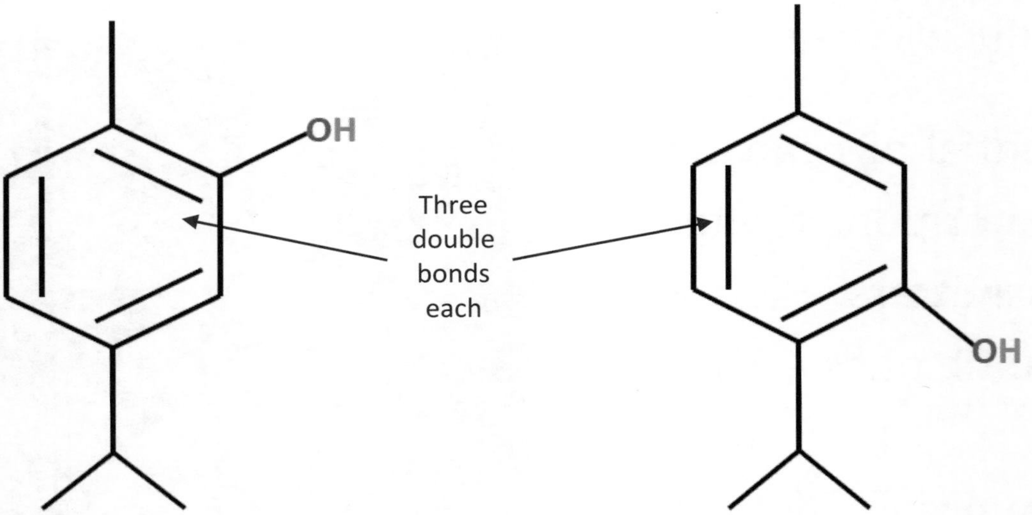

OH

Three
double
bonds
each

OH

Oil of Oregano
Carvacrol
$C_{10}H_{14}O$

Oil of Thyme
Thymol
$C_{10}H_{14}O$

The only difference between these two compounds is where the hydroxyl radical (**OH**) is attached. They are both phenylpropanoids and isomers of one another.

Thyme oil is a very important oil because it is one of the strongest natural antiseptics. It is able to kill over 60 different strains of bacteria including the common cold and gum disease.

♦Bent Keys and their Smellable Differences

The two structures below are not isomers, but they do have very distinctive odors and along with the carvacrol and thymol, they are principal ingredients in essential oils.

Do you know why the **H** is in front of the **O** in this structure?

Remember back to our discussion about valences? We learned that **oxygen** likes to hold onto two friends and **hydrogen** likes to hold onto one. Well if the **H** was on the inside, the **O** would not be able to grab on because the **H** would already be holding onto the **carbon** ring.

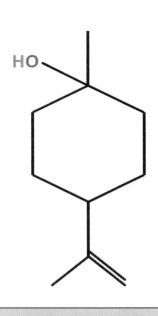

Tea Tree Oil
Terpinen-1-ol-4
$C_{10}H_{18}O$

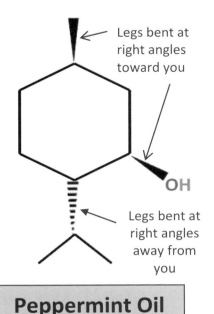

Legs bent at right angles toward you

OH

Legs bent at right angles away from you

Peppermint Oil
Menthol
$C_{10}H_{20}O$

The menthol molecule has no double bonds.

The main difference between the other three molecules that are shown and menthol is that menthol's top and bottom legs are bent. This creates a big difference in its smell.

75

♦Natural vs. Synthetic Menthol

The chemical formula for menthol is $C_{10}H_{20}O$. There are actually 19 known isomers of this formula, but we will only compare and contrast natural and synthetic isomers so you can understand how drug companies will take a natural product and create a synthetic one.

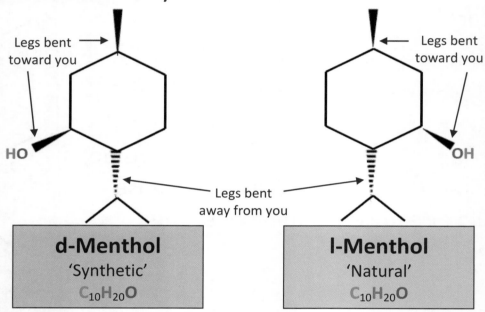

All menthols produced by living peppermint plants are left handed or levorotatory (l-menthol). They have a sharp, piercing, cold odor that is great for helping to clear congestion.

The right handed or dextrorotatory version of menthol is created in a laboratory with a slightly woody smell. It does not have any decongesting properties or the correct keys to let it into cellular receptor sites.

♦Blank Molecular Master Keys

When you need to have a new house key made you go to the hardware store and ask the clerk for assistance. He will ask to see your master key and find a blank template to match it to and then cut it to fit the original. This process can also be completed with a molecular blank key.

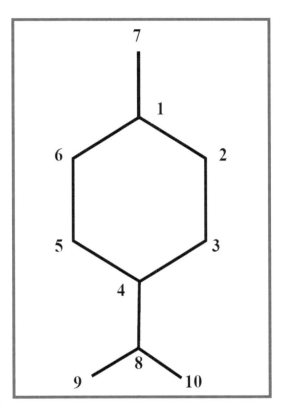

This shape is a blank master key for numerous essential oil molecules that act like chemical keys called ligands. These ligands sing their way to specific receptor sites of the cells. Scientists have numbered each of the carbon sites to identify the atoms. These numbers are incorporated into the scientific names of organic compounds. They identify where the oxygen, methyl, hydroxyl or propyl groups are attached.

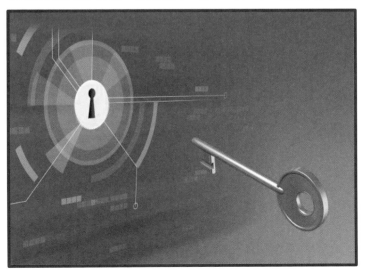

◆Essential Oil Species

Essential oils made from a single plant species can contain 100 to 400 different chemical compounds and many of those are trace elements.

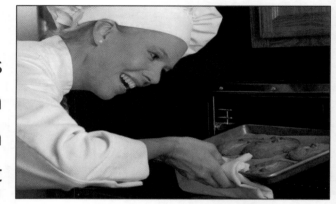

Due to all those trace elements there has never been an essential oil that has been completely analyzed; we just don't have sophisticated enough equipment yet. Therefore, scientists don't have the ability to recreate a complete essential oil in a laboratory. Chemists have yet to find all of the ingredients in even one species.

Imagine if a baker tried to recreate the most delicious chocolate chip cookie recipe ever, but did not know all the ingredients. He would not know that a special vanilla extract was the ingredient that made the cookies spectacular.

This is the same premise for essential oils. Chemists can try and recreate what God created, but without his talent, power, and expertise of all things they will not be able to account for all the ingredients in an oil and the oil won't work in the same healing way.

◆Trying to Map an Oil's Composition

Here are two examples of attempts to determine the chemical compounds in essential oils.

Orange Oil
(Citrus sinensis)

Chemists have

so far found:

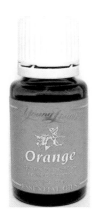

- 36 terpenoids
- 34 alcohols
- 30 esters
- 20 aldehydes
- 14 ketones
- 10 carboxylic acids
- flavonoids
- carotenoids
- steroids
- coumarins
- saccharides

They have found 15 known constituents, but suspect there may be as many as 200 additional compounds that cannot yet be identified.

Lavender Oil
(Lavandula angustifolia)

Chemists have

so far found:

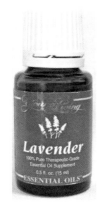

- 50 monoterpenes
- 10 sesquiterpenes
- 10-15 alcohols
- 10-15 esters
- 5 oxides
- 5 aldehydes
- 5 ketones
- 5 lactones

Scientists have identified 200 compounds, but believe they have only found half of all the constituents contained in lavender essential oil.

♦Botanical Families

Essential oils are complex living organisms created from a variety of plants. Plants are classified into broad categories according to common visual characteristics. These classifications are called *"families"*. There are hundreds of families and each family has a common name and a Latin name. The name of the family is capitalized and typically ends in 'ae.

The most common families of essential oil producing plants are in the table to the right: (see Stewart chapter eight for details).

The **mint family** has the most variations in oil compositions within the same species.

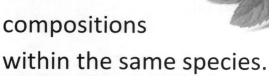

Latin Family Name	Common Family Name
Annonaceae	Ylang Ylang
Apiaceae	Celery/Carrot/Parsley
Araceae	Cane
Asteraceae	Aster/Daisy
Ericaceae	Heather
Burseraceae	Frankincense/Myrrh
Cistaceae	Cistus
Cupressaceae	Cypress
Geraniaceae	Geranium
Gramineae	Grass
Lamiaceae	**Mint** see table➔
Lauraceae	Laurel
Malvaceae	Hibiscus
Myristicaceae	Nutmeg
Myrtaceae	Myrtle
Oleaceae	Olive
Pinaceae	Pine
Piperaceae	Pepper
Rosaceae	Rose
Rutaceae	Citrus
Valerianaceae	Valerian
Zingiberaceae	Ginger

♦Mint Family Members that Produce Oil

Remember that common visual characteristics are what defines a plant's family, not the way it tastes or smells. So when you hear mint you

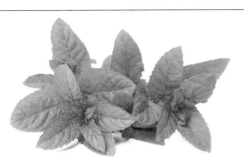

probably think of *'breath mint'* or *'minty mouthwash'*, but not all flavors of mints are actually in the mint family. Wintergreen is a common flavor of mints and gum, but is not a mint family member.   Oil producing members of the Mint Family are in the table below:

Mint Family Member	Latin Genus and Species
Basil	*Ocimum basilicum*
Clary Sage	*Salvia sclarea*
Hyssop	*Hyssopus officinalis*
Lavandin	*Lavandula x hybrid*
Lavender	*Lavandula angustifolia*
Marjoram	*Origanum marjorana*
Melissa	*Melissa officinalis*
Mountain Savory	*Satureja montana*
Oregano	*Origanum compactum*
Patchouli	*Pogostemon cablin*
Pennyroyal	*Mentha pulegium*
Peppermint	*Mentha piperita*
Rosemary	*Rosemarinus officinalis*
Sage	*Salvia officinalis*
Spearmint	*Mentha spicata*
Spike Lavender	*Lavandula latifolia*
Thyme	*Thymus vulgaris*
Vitex	*Vitex negundo*

The scientific names are always written in Latin. The first name is the 'genus' and is always capitalized. The last name is the 'species' and is always written in lower case.

A genus of the plant kingdom is also a broad category of plants.

♦Same Genus...Different Species

Genus: Lavandula

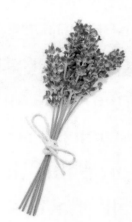

Members of this genus all have lavender-like fragrances because of high levels of the compounds linalool and linalyl acetate.   There are also differences like the extent of camphor that is or isn't present.

Lavandin

(*Lavandula x hybrid*)

Lavender

(*Lavandula augustifolio*)

Spike Lavender

(*Lavandula latifolia*)

Genus: Origanum

The two members of this genus that are listed can be used in place of one another, especially for a spicy pizza favoring, because they both contain y-terpinene. However, the therapeutic benefits differ greatly.

Oregano has phenolic carvacrol and is a hot oil while Marjoram contains terpinen-4-ol which makes it a gentle oil.

Oregano

(*Origanum compactum*)

Marjoram

(*Origanum marjorana*)

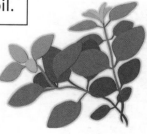

♦Seeds define the Species

The kind of seed is what determines the species of the plant. You cannot grow spike lavender from a lavender seed nor can you grow lavandin from a lavender seed.

Mature plants produce seeds much like human mothers produce babies. They have the same genetic characteristics as the parent. This genetic recipe is coded into the DNA of the plant and is consistent from crop to crop from year to year.

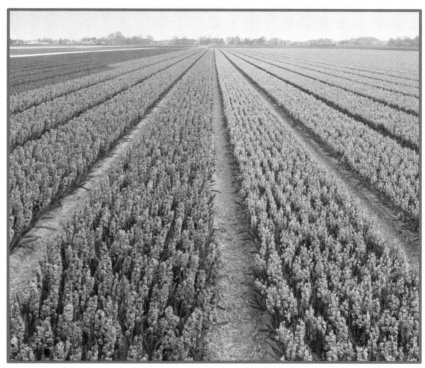

The essential oils from these plants are the same each year except for minor variations that happen because of the changes in rainfall, the amount of sun, or the location in which the seeds were planted. Some plants can be planted in different environments, adapt, and grow, but some cannot. Frankincense can only grow in the hot, dry regions of Arabia or Africa and no other place.

♦Seasonal Variations = Chemotypes

Seeds planted from the same species in different geographic locations can result in oils with different chemical make-ups. These variations are called chemotypes.

The chemotypes of oils cannot simply be described by their genus and species; they have to be labeled with the region in which the seeds are grown.

Many plants produce more essential oils at a certain time of the day: morning, afternoon, or evening. Other plants produce more oils at certain times of the year. Growers must have this knowledge to know when is the best time to harvest.

The essential oils in balsam fir trees act as an antifreeze and are the most potent in the middle of winter. Winter is the best time to harvest and distill the oil.

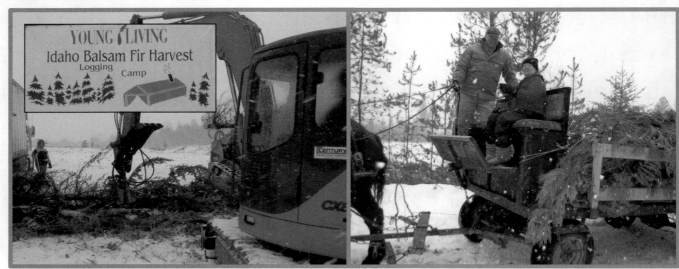

♦Chemotypes of Thyme

Let's take a packet of Thyme (*Thymus vulgaris*) seeds and plant them in different regions:

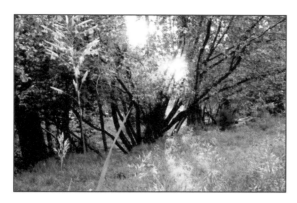

Thymol CT is cultivated in valleys and used in raindrop. It is harvested in the fall and is strongly antiseptic and aggressive to the skin.

Linalol CT is grown at high altitudes and is gentle and soothing. It provides a hostile environment for fungi and parasites.

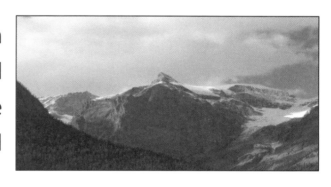

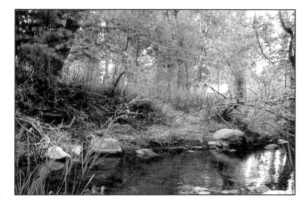

Thujanol CT is only found in the wild and shows no seasonal variations. When cultivated it shows a different chemotype. It is hormonally balancing.

Other Thymus vulgaris CTs are: Carvacrol; α-Terpineol; Geraniol; 1.8 Cineole; p-Cymene; and Phenol.

See Chemistry of Essential Oils Made Simple, by Stewart pages 240-251 for more on Species and Chemotypes

◆Essential Oils vs. Pharmaceuticals

As stated on the previous pages, each batch of essential oils differ ever so slightly due to the variations in growing (sun, rain, soil composition, etc.).

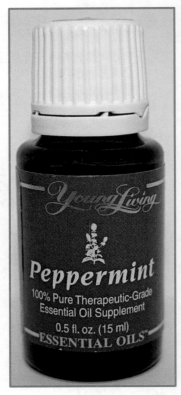

It is specifically these natural variations that allow essential oils to be so effective in providing hostile environments to microbes, viruses, bacteria, and other harmful things that try to invade our bodies.

Due to this natural variation of essential oils the microbes, viruses, and bacteria cannot mutate and change to avoid being killed by the essential oils. However, this is not the same with pharmaceuticals created in a lab. By

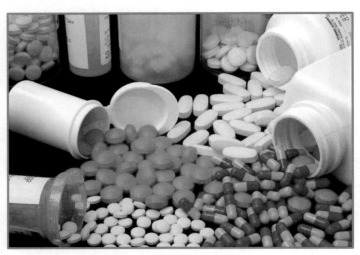

law, the formula of the patented drug must be the same each and every time. Therefore, microbes, viruses, and bacteria have the opportunity to mutate and become drug resistant.

♦Chemistry of an Oil is More than DNA

The exact chemistry of an essential oil goes beyond genetic code and has much to do with how an oil is grown and the way it was cultivated and harvested. Finally, the manner in which it was extracted and distilled also impacts the final essential oil product.

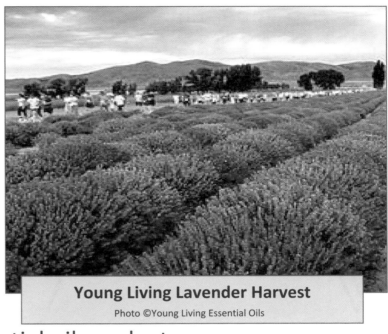

Young Living Lavender Harvest
Photo ©Young Living Essential Oils

Key Considerations of an Essential Oil

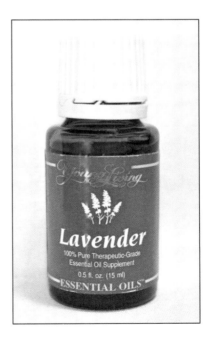

- Chemical composition is predetermined by genetic codes in the seeds.
- Genus and species are required to identify the plant.
- Chemotypes are environmentally dependent.
- Harvesting time of day, year, etc. impacts oil composition.
- Chemotype is to essential oils what vintage is to wine.
- Growing conditions outsmart germs.

♦Isoprene Units

The most important compound in essential oils is called an 'Isoprene' and people say it looks like a horse or a chair.

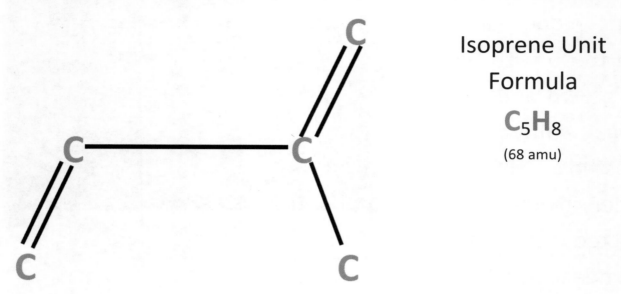

Isoprene Unit
Formula
C_5H_8
(68 amu)

Remember that each carbon (**C**) has a valence of four so there are hydrogens (**H**) completing each molecule.

Can you count the hydrogens to add-up to 8?

The picture above is never shown. Instead, the **C** atoms are implied at each angle, at convergence of lines, and at the end of each line.

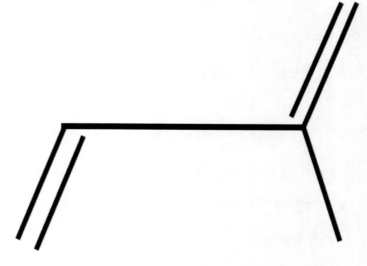

♦Isoprenes as Building Blocks

The isoprene unit is the building block from which all essential oils are made. In fact, this unit is the most frequently found functional group in the living tissues of animals and plants on earth.

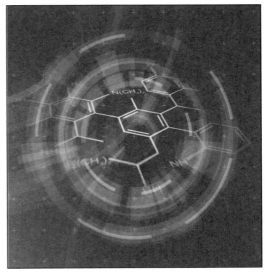

Molecules built using isoprenes are called 'terpenoids'. To make these terpenoid molecules, isoprenes link up in two ways: (1) in chains and (2) in rings.

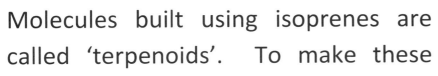

- ♦ **Acyclic** (Chains like lycopene or myrcene)
  - ○ Example: isoprene units in a chain
- ♦ **Cyclic** (rings in the structure)
  - ○ Example: isoprene units in a ring
- ♦ **Monocyclic** = 1 ring (carvacrol, furan, or carvone)
- ♦ **Bicyclic** = 2 rings (umbelliferone or sabinene)
- ♦ **Tricyclic** = 3 rings (bergaptene or psoralen)

The isoprene units just keep connecting together and getting larger and heavier.

◆Terpenes

Terpenes are the most common class of compounds found in essential oils. Two isoprenes combined create a terpene and is called a 'terpene unit'. They are simple hydrocarbons until they become oxygenated.

There are classes of terpenes found in essential oils classified by the number of isoprenes and weight.

Name	Terpene Units	Formula	Molecular Weight
Monoterpene	1	$C_{10}H_{16}$	163
Sesquiterpenes	1.5	$C_{15}H_{24}$	204
Diterpene	5	$C_{20}H_{32}$	272
Triterpene	3	$C_{30}H_{48}$	408
Tetraterpene	4	$C_{40}H_{64}$	544

Essential oils are composed of very tiny molecules and the above terpenes are the only ones you will find in distilled essential oils.

There is a green line under the triterpenes because molecules larger than 500 amu will not get through the distillation process nor through human skin or blood-brain barrier.

> **Fun Fact:** There are an estimated 1,000 different monoterpenes and more than 3,000 sesquiterpenes found in essential oils!

⬥Essential Oils and PMS

Dr. Stewart popularized the "PMS Theory" to explain how essential oils can work together like a good soccer team. Essentially, it starts with a good line-up.

⬥**P** =   Phenols (*or Phenylpropanoids*)

⬥**M** = Monoterpenes

⬥**S** =   Sesquiterpenes

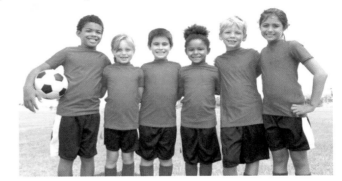

Then each player must have a specific position to play:

⬥**P** =   Phenols are the starting line; they get into the cells and clean the receptor sites like new.

⬥**S** =   Sesquiterpenes then head to those sparkling clean receptors and delete any bad information that is being stored there, such as disease.

⬥**M** = Monoterpenes are the third wave; they head in and restore or awaken the correct information from the cells' DNA.

This PMS Theory can be a useful in helping to give us guidance for mixing and applying therapeutic grade essential oils in an effective way to provide the body with tools to heal itself.

"Let's express it another way:

1) When cellular intercommunication is restored in the body by clean, well-functioning receptor sites,

2) When garbled or miswritten information in the cellular job description has been erased,

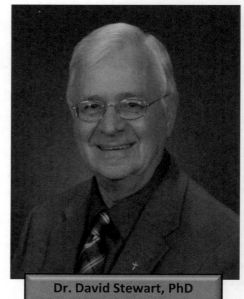

Dr. David Stewart, PhD

3) When God's image of perfection, that has always been there in the field of the cell from our creation, has been revived and re-installed, then whatever our disease or condition has been, the conditions for its presence does not exist anymore.

Our disease or condition was the consequence of miscommunications between cells and erroneous information within the cells that caused them to malfunction. When these basic errors have been corrected, as is possible with **P**[*phenolics*] **M**[*monoterpenes*] **S**[*sesquiterpenes*], the problem disappears. It can take time, like days, weeks, or months, but it can also be instantaneous." (Stewart, pg. 292).

Note: the words phenols and phenolics are interchangeable

♦PMS in Raindrop Technique

Raindrop technique is a sequence of applying essential oils to the feet and back that involves various ancient techniques. It was developed by D. Gary Young, N.D. and is a powerfully effective healing modality and anointing procedure.

The oils used in Raindrop Technique create a perfect PMS Anointing.

Oil	Phenols (*Cleanse*)	Monoterpenes (*Restore*)	Sesquiterpenes (*Erase*)
Valor	8%	54%	4%
Oregano	72%	18%	4%
Thyme	58%	37%	3%
Basil	77%	3%	0%
Wintergreen	97%	0%	0%
Marjoram	37%	44%	4%
Cypress	8%	76%	14%
Peppermint	63%	10%	9%
Weighted Oil Averages	44%	35%	5%

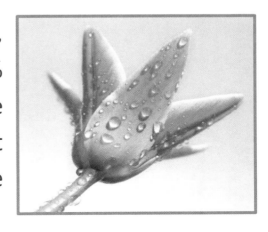

The average PMS oil is 44% phenols, 35% monoterpenes, and 5% sesquiterpenes. If you look at the averages in the table you will see that marjoram is the closest to the 'perfect PMS oil'.

◆The Raindrop Oils

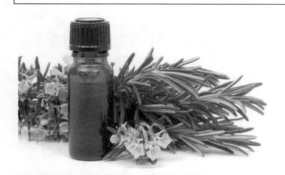

Each of the essential oils in the Raindrop Technique was chosen for its specific components and how it affects the body.

Oil	Description
Valor®	Gentle and soothing, balances the body electrically, enhances feelings of confidence, courage, and self-esteem.
Oregano	One of the most powerful antimicrobial essential oils, may help with colds, digestion, and to balance the metabolism.
Thyme	Immune enhancing, supports the body's natural defenses, and can help supply energy under stress.
Basil	Muscle relaxing to voluntary and involuntary muscles, mentally energizing and invigorating.
Wintergreen	Supports joints and skeletal structure, cortisone-like effect, with analgesic properties like aspirin.
Marjoram	Relaxing and calming to muscles, promotes peace and sleep, may help anxiety.
Cypress	Supports the circulatory and lymphatic systems, beneficial for asthma, and colds.
Peppermint	Supports digestive, respiratory, and nervous systems. Used for headaches and improves concentration and mental retention.
AromaSiez®	Calming, relaxing, and relieves tension. Relaxes muscles and may relieve headaches.

⬥Cleanliness is next to Godliness

The raindrop oils are mostly cleansing compounds; therefore, it is easy to see why the raindrop technique is such a powerful detoxifier. It cleans receptor sites and gets rid of the toxins at all levels in every organ and every tissue of the body.

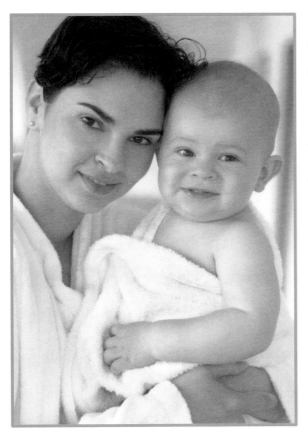

Ancient Hebrew writings teach us that "Cleanliness is next to Godliness." This not only applies to the outside of our bodies, but the inside too. We must achieve and maintain our health. When we use essential oils to cleanse our bodies at a cellular level we are maintaining our bodily temple. That is the benefit of the raindrop technique.

Oils are complex substances that have many healing properties. Raindrop is just one of the ways to get essential oils into the body, but it is a powerful one!

♦What is Raindrop?

Raindrop Technique was created by D. Gary Young in the 1980's through his practice, research, and development of therapeutic grade essential oils.

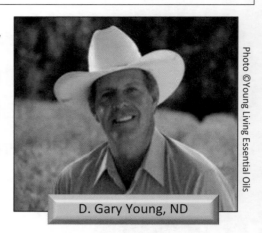

D. Gary Young, ND

Photo ©Young Living Essential Oils

The technique is called 'Raindrop' because seven single oils and two oil blends are dropped from a height of six inches onto the back like drops of rain. This is combined with Ancient Tibetan Vita Flex and Native American feathering techniques. The oils start to penetrate the body instantly to bring it back into structural and electrical alignment.

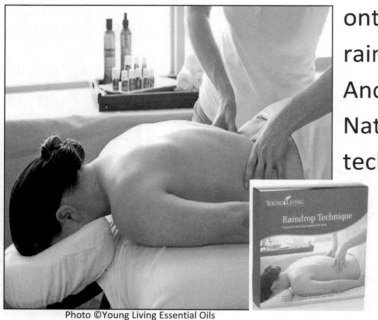

Photo ©Young Living Essential Oils

This process is based on the French model for applying oils which is the most extensively practiced and studied medicinal model in the world using oils.

⬥Wrap-up about Essential Oils

This book has been distilled (*pun intended!*) from the wonderful text "The Chemistry of Essential Oils Made Simple" by David Stewart, Ph.D., D.N.M.

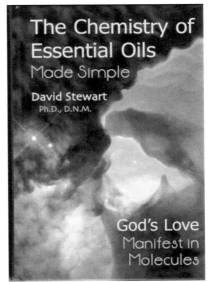

Part one includes 508 pages of text and 203 pages of tables that break down the compounds of essential oils into easy to understand lists.

Part two is a catalog of compounds in essential oils in easy to read table format.

Part three of the book goes "Beyond Chemistry" and into Quantum Physics and adds an additional 125 pages of reading material.

Some of the most helpful information regarding essential oils in the book is in chapter twelve:

- Plastic
- Clockwise activation
- Carrier oils
- More or less
- Oil safety

- Heat and light
- Shelf life
- Skin
- Allergies
- X-rays

Happy and Safe Oiling! *Michelle*

♦Resources

♦Reading

- Chemistry of Essential Oils Made Simple (Stewart)
- Essential Oils Desk Reference (ESP)
- Reference Guide for Essential Oils (Higley)
- Essential Oils Integrative Medical Guide (Young)
- Vibrational Raindrop Technique (Bonds-Garrett)
- Healing Oils of the Bible (Stewart)
- Healing for the Age of Enlightenment (Burrows)
- Statistical Validation of Raindrop Technique (Stewart)

♦Essential Oils

For more information about Young Living Essential Oils, please contact Independent Distributor Michelle Truman (#29348) at www.truessentials.net or 702-468-4162.

♦Classes

Michelle teaches classes at her center **Truessentials: The Center for Aromatherapy Education in Las Vegas** on Raindrop Technique, Applied Vitaflex, Oils of Scripture, Emotional Releasing with Essential Oils, and Chemistry of Essential Oils. See www.truessentials.net for additional classes by Michelle or www.RaindropTraining.com.

About the Author

Michelle M. Truman, Ed.D., F.C.C.I. has been in the field of education since she graduated from Southern Utah University in the spring of 1995. She started working as a public school teacher that fall. She earned her Master's Degree in Curriculum and Instruction from University of Nevada, Las Vegas in 1998 with an emphasis in reading and literacy. In 2003 she earned her Doctoral Degree in Curriculum and Instruction with an emphasis in writing, cultural studies, and teacher development.

In 1996 Michelle was introduced to essential oils through her parents, but was the type of oiler that you could classify as using the oils as a 'First Aid Kit'. That type of oil usage went on until 2008 until she attended her first CARE (Center for Aromatherapy Research and Education) Intensive class. Dr. Truman was amazed at how much there was to learn about the oils and how they could benefit her family in a much deeper way than just being a 'First Aid' source.

Dr. Truman became a Certified CARE Instructor in 2010 and opened Truessentials: The Center for Aromatherapy Education in Las Vegas in 2012. She also serves as an instructor for the Natural Therapies Certification Board and is a Certified Aromatherapy Coach and a Licensed Spiritual Health Coach. She enjoys reading, researching, and writing books. She is married with two grown daughters who are both oilers.

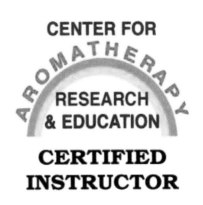